Eye Won

[POWERFULLY POSITIVE,
RIDICULOUSLY RESILIENT]

INCLUDES BONUS INTERACTIVE BOOK

Eye Won

[POWERFULLY POSITIVE, RIDICULOUSLY RESILIENT]

Jess Van Zeil

First published in 2019 by Dean Publishing
PO Box 119
Mt. Macedon, Victoria, 3441
Australia
deanpublishing.com

DEAN
PUBLISHING

Copyright © Jessica Van Zeil
jessvanzeil.com

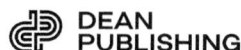

Cataloguing-in-Publication Data
National Library of Australia
Title: Eye Won: Powerfully Positive, Ridiculously Resilient
Edition: 1st edn
ISBN: 978-1-9254521-6-7
Category: Autobiography/Self-help

This is an autobiography, the author has tried to recreate events, locales and conversations from her memories of them. In order to maintain anonymity of certain individuals in some instances names, occupations and places have been changed to protect individuals. Certain identifying characteristics and details such as physical properties, occupations and places of residence may have changed.

This book is a personal memoir and not intended as a substitute for the medical advice of physicians. The reader should regularly consult a physician in matters relating to his/her health and particularly with respect to any symptoms that may require diagnosis or medical attention. This is not intended for medical purposes or promote any particular type of treatment than that recommended to the individual from their own medical team— each person is different.

The views and opinions expressed in this book are those of the authors and do not necessarily reflect the official policy or position of any other agency, publisher, organization, employer or company. Assumptions made in the analysis are not reflective of the position of any entity other than the author(s) — and, these views are always subject to change, revision, and rethinking at any time.

The authors or organizations are not to be held responsible for misuse, reuse, recycled and cited and/or uncited copies of content within this book by others.

DEDICATION

To my parents, without you I would not be the woman I
am today and none of this would be possible.

CONTENTS

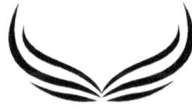

INTRODUCTION

I was born in South Africa — the "rainbow nation" of diversity, home to many languages, cultures and creeds. Life for my siblings and I was bursting with adventure and filled with laughter, love, family and friends. Idyllic really.

I was loved by my family and my extended family, in particular my "African mum" Dora; a beautiful and kind woman who had worked with my family since my own mum's youth. Trips to Kruger National Park were both unforgettable and regular occurrences; the majesty of wild lions, leopards, elephants and giraffes showed me the wonder and vibrancy of life that seemed to seep into my soul.

I spent a lot of time with my grandparents in a small town on the south coast. Granny Annie indulged me for hours of play in make-believe games all summer long. Her beautiful, love-filled face, soft skin and snow-white hair filled the corners of my heart and she always accepted me just as I was.

I remember one day when I was staying at my grandparents on the coast, I found a piece of old lace curtain that Granny was going to throw away. It was such a beautiful flowy piece of white lace that I instantly saw wings in the wind. I couldn't believe anyone could throw something so marvellous away.

I grabbed the shred of lace and started dancing, skipping and running through the garden. It was magical and made me feel effortlessly beautiful. Granny watched from the balcony, amused by my innocent joy and love for a tatty old curtain.

Eventually she called out intrigued as to what I was pretending to be.

"Are you a bird, my Jessie?"

I stopped in my tracks, a bird?! Couldn't she see?

"I'm a princess, fairy-ish, sort of snow-white, tinkerbell-ish," I said as if it were blatantly obvious and continued dancing around her garden for hours. Granny sat back laughing at her quirky five-year-old granddaughter. Perhaps it was an early warning sign of a girl that wanted to do, see and experience it — and all at once. In her own magical way.

Her love for me and my quirky ways were a match made in heaven.

But behind the fairy-dust of the lace curtain, growing up in South Africa could be both beautiful and brutal, our daily life could also be constantly tinged with danger. I was always surrounded by massive three-metre-high walls covered in barbed wire and electric fencing on top; not to keep me in, but rather to keep the bad people out. As I grew, I learned that armed burglary was a constant threat and worry; I would have nightmares about it.

Our family home had been broken into at least five times and everyone had a tale of warning to share about armed intruders, stolen property or even shootings. I was exposed to significant poverty and scarcity. Beggars were commonplace and the effects of alcoholism and addiction were everywhere even though I didn't fully understand the afflictions themselves. I remained quite protected by the shelter of the private girls' school I attended and the strict but fair lessons of the nuns. My parents did everything to shield me from trouble and protect me from danger.

For all the adventure I experienced, and all the love I was surrounded by, we missed the deep-seated peace in our lives.

My beloved Dora became a victim of the AIDS epidemic; the shame, social adversity and ultimately the deep loss was cruel. I was so lost and confused. I asked when Dora would be better so I could kiss her again, I was told she would never be better again. That was the knowledge we had back then and it tore at my young heart.

My parents' dream to give us everything forged a move to Australia. Though I was still a child, this decision angered and hurt me as I was very happy with my life and deep down was afraid of leaving loved ones behind, of moving and the change that awaited me.

Their application to Australia was accepted when I was eight years old. We soon landed on foreign soil. The picturesque southern suburbs of Melbourne and the familiar smell of the seaside reminded me of our seaside holidays with my grandparents which made me feel more at home. As we drove along, there wasn't a sky-high fence in sight, there were kids riding their bikes down the street, not an adult to be seen! My parents seemed to relax immediately, as though the fear they'd been holding onto their entire lives had finally been released.

I quickly fell in love with the freedom of riding around the block, playing in my garden without my parents' hovering eyes. I was always gallivanting outside, playing sports or organising a crab-hunt at the beach!

I distinctly remember being rather underwhelmed when I saw my first koala at the zoo. Having wild African animals as your benchmark leaves anything else a bit tame by comparison!

There were a few unexpected hurdles, like the day my parents explained I'd be going to a co-ed school – BOYS? I had a meltdown; I had traumatic memories from South Africa where games of kiss-chasey with grubby preschool boys meant sloppy unwanted kisses. However, within weeks of starting my new school I was kicking footy with the boys and happily running around the schoolyard. Luckily, girls at this school had 'cooties' and boys didn't wrestle them for kisses.

This foreign country had truly begun to feel like home.

In a way, the new independence suited my soul. I'd always liked to play by my own rules and adventure beyond 'the norm'. The new freedom breathed more life into my cheeky nature and gave me more reason to push boundaries.

It was such a relief when I discovered that Australia was a sports-obsessed country. I loved playing all types of sports and quickly adapted to kicking a footy and playing a large variety of sports, in particular Judo.

My teenage years were relatively typical in terms of trying to keep up with my friends, fashions and trends. Boys became more than mere team mates on the sporting field and I found myself diving deeper into my own life to avoid my parent's marital troubles.

Though Mum and Dad remained my rocks in life, my pillars of strength. I was determined to live by my rules. I had an insatiable appetite for living and surrounded myself in adventure, dreams and ambition.

Granny, who migrated to Australia two years after us, always reminded me to look at what I did have in life, not what I didn't have. Though I always loved my angelic Granny, I used to roll my eyes and think her point was an outdated way of thinking; that she'd never understand what it was like to be a teenager in the 21st century. Her "adopt an attitude of gratitude" mantra was sweet but archaic. The brattier I became, the more attitude and eye-rolls I served up, and the more persistent Granny became with her gratitude message.

When I was 20 years old, Granny brought every single one of her grandkids a little journal and asked us to write one thing every day that we were grateful for or that made us smile. I did it, not because I believed it would help me in anyway, not because I thought it would change my life, but because I knew it would make Granny smile, and that was worth writing in this silly little journal.

Little did I know the role gratitude would end up playing in my life. That it would become a lifeline during the turbulent times that were soon approaching. That Mum and Dad, my siblings, my grandparents and Granny's ritual of counting blessings — would soon be the buoy I would cling to as life's rugged sea came crashing down and into my life.

I sometimes wonder whether life prepares us in advance for things that may happen. Not everyone is lucky enough to have a happy childhood, loving parents and siblings, kind grandparents and live in a free country. I had them all. Though it certainly wasn't all sunshine and rainbows, it was mine. And I loved my life in its eclectic tapestry of events and experiences.

If there was one thing I had discovered in my first two decades of life, it was that life was to be lived. And I planned to do it well. Very well indeed. Dreams swarmed my mind with enthusiasm. And I planned on chasing them.

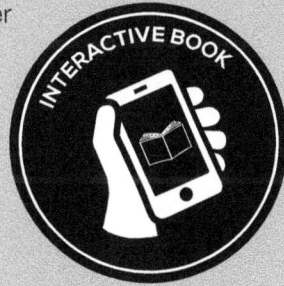

Jess is sharing so much more in her INTERACTIVE book.

See exclusive, behind-the-scenes videos, audios and photos of Jess's journey.

DOWNLOAD free content and learn how to become powerfully positive and ridiculously resilient.

deanpublishing.com/eyewon

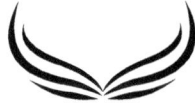

CHAPTER 1

THE "C" WORD

"I only do what my gut tells me to. I think it's smart to listen to other people's advice, but at the end of the day, you're the only one who can tell you what's right for you."
— *Jennifer Lopez*

Here I was, twenty years old and falling in love with my life. It was October 2013 and I had nearly completed my first year of university studying nutrition. I loved combining my love of sport with the science of health. I had incredible friends, work that I enjoyed, exciting holidays planned for the upcoming summer break; I was living my dreams.

As my exams approached, I noticed that the harmless looking spot on my left eye had begun to deepen in colour and irritate my eye. The GP said it would probably have to be lasered off and that was my expectation when I innocently went along to an appointment with a local ophthalmologist. My friend Gemma drove me, as I didn't think it would take long.

Boy was I wrong! Two hours later I had gone from room to room completing a series of tests on the front and back of my eyes, on my vision and had photographs taken of every millimetre of both eyes.

After analysing the results, the doctor abruptly explained what he wanted done.

"We need to remove the spot and complete a biopsy on the tissue. This needs to be done as soon as possible; there's a small chance it's cancer – I don't think it is – but just to be safe."

My mind exploded! Did he just use the dreaded 'C' word? Cancer? There's no way! I'm so young – I felt fine!

The doctor didn't notice my reaction; he just kept talking about some other minor irregularity he'd detected, but I was lost in the heavy buzzing sound that had started in my head. I could barely respond; swamped with the awful possibility that this harmless spot could be cancer.

Somewhere in his lecture, I found myself objecting, *"But I don't have private health insurance."* He warned me sharply that if I decided to use the public system it would take six months just to get an appointment.

His clipped words continued ominously, *"If this is cancer you don't have that kind of time to play with."* I couldn't connect the words he was saying with his dismissive tone. How could he dump the weight of the word cancer on me like that?!

I felt faint as the implications swam around my head. How would I explain this to my parents – that it could be cancer? That it cost $1700 for private surgery? Things were already tight; I thought they'd be mad!

He could fit me in for surgery two days after my exams but I would have to let him know quick-smart. I was terrified and felt so trapped by his words. In a daze, I arranged a follow-up appointment. Aside from making me feel that I didn't matter, that I was just dollar signs sitting on the seat in front of him; that cold, indifferent doctor, Dr Moneybags, had me utterly freaked out!

On the drive home, Gemma was left dumbfounded too. It was the first time I had to say the words, *"I might have cancer."*

That night was even worse. Mum wanted so much information that I either just didn't know or wanted to forget. Her face crumpled in devastation when I dropped the 'C' word. Her next reaction took me by surprise, *"Well we just have to do it; we don't have another option!"*

I objected quickly, *"But we can't afford it!"*

Mum looked surprised, *"Jess, your life is worth more to me than any amount of money!"* Those were both the best and the worst words I could have hoped for! Her words reassured me of her unfailing support but they also highlighted that my life may actually be on the line.

Dad was still in South Africa. My parents' marriage had fallen apart a few years previously, and he had moved back to his homeland to do some soul searching. While the relationships between us all went through some pretty tumultuous times, the bond of family was forever strong and my dad's reaction was immediate. He insisted he would be back in Australia before my next appointment. He needed to hear from Dr Moneybags himself. *How can it cost that much and why? If he thinks it is cancer why is Moneybags being so flippant?*

I didn't know the answers. I had no clue why this potential threat that was looming over my head and impacting the lives of my family and friends, why it was all being so easily dismissed by this doctor.

Days after, I was utterly lost and consumed in my own head. My mind kept repeating what the doctor had said – cancer – cost – decide! I'm glad he didn't diagnose it yet so I couldn't google it relentlessly! The only thing I accomplished was totally ignoring the study I should have been doing for my exams.

Dad's presence at the next appointment gave me someone to lean on. When the doctor asked what I had decided for the surgery, I was bewildered. Thankfully, Actionman Dad stepped in with a truckload of questions. One of those questions *"Why has this happened? What has occurred to change this from a burst blood vessel to a potential cancer threat?"*

This became the common go-to question my parents, friends and even the media asked, as they all looked for something to blame.

Dr Moneybags blandly replied, *"I can't tell you why a nevus* (fancy word for a mole) *one day becomes malignant* (cancerous) *... but even if it is cancer, don't worry, it's easily fixed with surgery. You'll be on chemotherapy eye-drops for a year or two and that will be it."*

We were both shocked by his arrogance and complete disregard for the emotional turmoil that goes alongside cancer.

Though most health professionals I've met on this journey have been fabulous kind-hearted people, the insensitive ones certainly stand out in my memory too.

Although we felt unsure and confused by Dr Moneybag's demeanour, one thing he made clear; we couldn't waste time: we signed the surgery agreement and left. Though I had signed the medical document, this whole saga was not something I'd signed up for in my life.

~ My First Surgery ~

In a haze, I trudged through my exams, jumbled thoughts swirling around, unable to articulate everything I had learnt that semester. After each exam, I was tormented with feelings of failure. I would be lucky to even pass. The lead up was incredibly draining with migraines and sleepless nights; I was dreading it.

So instead of celebrating the end of exams, I had to prepare for surgery. I hate early mornings, especially the fasting kind. No food? No COFFEE! But rules are rules, so as that Friday dawned, I begrudgingly put on the ugly surgery gown and Dad helped me nervously climb into the clinical surgery bed. White clinical, cold sheets weren't much of a comfort.

I would be the first patient to be operated on due to my latex allergy – this is something I was grateful for as I meant I was not only first but the environment would be at its most sterile.

People fussed around me; the wonderful anaesthetist reassured me that I'd soon be at home in bed. I squeezed Dad's hand and said goodbye as they rolled me into theatre.

Waking up groggy and disorientated wasn't pleasant; a hot, dry mouth with noisy machines and nurses darting around me. That first cold sip of apple juice was heaven; I came to love that physical sensation post-surgery. I was keen to get home so I wobbled around in the change rooms, falling over putting my pants on, missing holes repeatedly. I was too stubborn to admit that I needed help. I didn't break any speed records but at least I dressed myself. Yep, putting on my own pants was quite the achievement.

With some painkillers and a pesky follow-up appointment in ten days' time, I made it home. Awaiting me was the biggest hamper of every sweet food your heart could desire arranged by the world's best mum. Mine. I'm sure the button of my jeans burst just by looking at all that chocolate – my recovery had begun!

Within days I was out socialising and soon after back working at the café. Everything felt pretty normal again despite the little underlying stress in the air as we waited for the biopsy results. I was both relieved and nervous when the appointment rolled around; at least we'll have our answer, but will it be the answer we want?

My parents came with me and to our surprise the histology came back as benign.

Thank god, I was cancer free! I had dodged a bullet. Learning how valuable life was and how quickly things could change. I was so grateful.

But then I felt this growing sense of guilt. We had made such a big deal out of this whole 'cancer' thing though it actually wasn't something to worry about. I had wasted my parents' hard-earned money for what? Peace of mind? Sure – that was great but we should have just waited a little and gone through the public system.

I was so angry at Dr Moneybags. He alarmed me into a position without options while in reality there were some. He was one cold, mean asshole, he wanted me to think I had cancer in order to line his back pocket. He used fear to bully me into using *him* instead of the public system. His name was fitting. Or should it be Dr Master Manipulator?

Had I known then what I know now, I would have got a second opinion. In fact, I'd urge anyone in moments of doubt and confusion to get a second opinion, to not be manipulated into a decision like I was.

I had another few check-ups with Dr Moneybags and was told I didn't need to come back for 6-12 months. I was not given a warning of potential regrowth. I was not warned that if it came back there was a high likelihood it would be cancerous. Something you'd think worth mentioning, hey?

I thought I had gotten away unscathed. Two months later, this whole "cancer scare episode" was over and I happily brushed my hands of it. Unfortunately, I wasn't so lucky with my university results. From my standing as a distinction student first semester; I had slunk to barely a pass in each subject. I was devastated, it wasn't a fail but it was close enough; I promised myself to work harder the following year. It made the top of my to-do list, I had to climb back to my usual level.

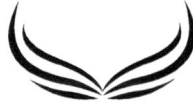

CHAPTER 2

REBOUND FROM SOUTH AFRICA

"Hope lies in dreams, in imagination, and in the courage of those who dare to make dreams into reality."

— *Jonas Salk*

Summertime ... my life post-surgery quickly returned to normal, a fabulous kinda normal.

I worked incredibly long hours in our busy beachside café but managed to sneak away for a beautiful family holiday on the gorgeous Merimbula beaches. Best of all, I revitalised myself by going skydiving. This was topped off by an adventure through Laos and Thailand with one of my best friends, Kathryn, just before the semester began. The cancer scare was a thing of the past, Jess was back in action, never wanting to miss an opportunity.

Between study, work and being involved in extra university groups, I was extremely busy but loving every minute of it, while looking ahead to making plans for my 21st birthday in July. However, more of my dreams were knocking at the door of my adventurous heart and I set my eyes on a trip to South Africa. Not just a conventional safari. Between November and July of the following year I would see the sights, undertake some volunteer work and most thrilling of all, complete one of my dreams of becoming a SCUBA diving instructor.

Gemma would join me for seven weeks of adventuring. I wouldn't abandon my studies altogether though and would return for the second semester in 2015. My family were not so enthusiastic about this plan of mine. Finish my degree they said, get a real job, be a grown-up; all that boring stuff!

One morning in June my heart sank. I noticed a few dark spots growing on my eye. I couldn't bear the thought of seeing Dr Moneybags again. I didn't need a repeat of his bullying and all the stress that it caused for nothing. I didn't need to hand him over extra cash so he could get richer.

I refused to let my university grades suffer the way it had the previous year, especially over another benign nevus thingy. To my mum's dismay I postponed the doctors until the end of October, after I had finished my exams. And I did really well! I completed everything I set out to do and I happily finished the academic year, eagerly looking towards South Africa.

However, those dark spots had been growing bigger every month. When my appointment rolled around, Dr Moneybags took one look at my left eye and started to panic, "You need to go and see another specialist ASAP!" His referral to a front-of-the-eye specialist was going to take a few weeks.

"That's not going to work I'm afraid; I'm leaving on an 8-month trip in 10 days."

He rebuffed me strongly, "You have to cancel it, or at least delay it until we work out what this is."

I scoffed at him; I still didn't trust him after the way he had disregarded my feelings yet was happy to take my money the year before. He may seem panicked now but there was no way I was changing my plans just because he said I should. I wouldn't be led down his pathway as easily as last time.

There was nothing Dr Moneybags could say to change my mind. I was determined to start my trip as planned, I couldn't delay it by another three months – let alone afford to! Everything was paid for; I had packed my bags – packed up my life! Eventually he saw my heels dug in and he realised that compromise was the only option. I was in charge. We agreed I could go as long as I saw a specialist in South Africa as soon as I got there. Done deal, Moneybags.

Relaying everything that night to Dad, he immediately organised an appointment with one of the best ophthalmologists in the country, two days after I arrived. I admit, I relaxed after hearing that. This doctor was the best around, so surely, he'd just take a look and send me on my way, or he'll perform a quick overnight surgery and let me keep living out my dream trip – sorted!

Mum and the rest of my family were not convinced. They thought this was too serious to have hanging over my head as I ran off overseas. I didn't realise how bad things could become. I was young and determined, my doctor had given me clearance to go, I had another appointment locked in so I couldn't see what all the fuss was about. I was fine!

I believed that I was somehow above cancer, I was twenty-one and felt like I owned the world; everything would be fine because I was strong and had so many dreams to live out! I remembered the early assurance that even if it were cancer; surgery and eye drops would send it packing, so it was simply the latest hurdle between freedom and me!

Mum was torn at me leaving but she knew my decision and graciously sent me off with a smile.

I was unbelievably excited; desperate to show Gemma around my beautiful homeland! I put the minor stress at the back of my mind, I'd jump that hurdle when it comes. For now, it's travel time.

~ Travelling Standby ~

Only in Africa could you have such a lavish feast as my family laid out for us when we arrived; every kind of meat imaginable cooked to perfection. Gem was welcomed with open arms and we had our own rooms at my uncle's house, we even had a car at our disposal.

Underneath this picture-perfect holiday, were many reasons why we weren't staying at my dad's place. At that time, I was still processing the countless emotions from him moving back to South Africa and also that he'd moved in with a new partner very soon after his separation from Mum.

At separate times I had felt denial, grief, hurt, abandonment and anger at him, without knowing how to process each of them. I certainly wasn't ready to stay with him and his new partner Ash. I thought it would be seen as forgiving him for all the hurt he had caused Mum and my siblings. I could only take our relationship one day at a time.

For a few days I could relax, get over the jetlag and prepare for our imminent road trip. I had that troublesome appointment to get out of the way first and so I went along to meet the ophthalmologist, Dr Sunnies. Dr Sunnies had an amazing collection of special sunglasses next to the reception desk. They were fun and colourful and every time I was in that waiting room I would try a different pair on.

Dr Sunnies didn't see it as straightforward as I did. He certainly did not like what he was looking at. He was worried enough to book me in for surgery the very next day.

I had almost convinced myself there would be another way forward other than urgent surgery. I was meant to be enjoying my trip, not running around stressing about this annoying thing on my eye! But then I realised the faster this operation was over the faster we could start travelling around. So, the plan was that I'd have urgent surgery and be on my way. Sure – no problem!

The surgery was booked in for the afternoon so I indulged in a three-course breakfast. Gem drove me to the doctors and simultaneously underwent a crash course of South Africa's traffic bedlam: road rules are mere guidelines that no one really follows. It's hard to describe the mayhem; hardly any cars are roadworthy; people drive on the nature strip, cut you off, travel at half the speed limit while others travel at double!

I was very impressed by the hospital; it was beautiful, comfortable and pristine with warm, relaxed nurses. Dad met us there and we waited for the process to begin. I wasn't nearly as nervous this time, I had a better idea of what the surgery entailed and I held a lot of trust in Dr Sunnies. He made me feel comfortable and in a way, I felt in control.

I was again groggy and bothersome to the nurses when I woke up. The fabulous taste of fresh juice pepped me up and I was at my uncle's and in bed before I knew it. I was exhausted but already starting to feel better and think clearly.

At the first check-up, I was direct, there was something I needed to know. Something important.

"When can we start our road trip?"

Dr Sunnies said I would have to wait a week – sure, I could do that. Have a few more check-ups too – sure. He was optimistic. He mentioned that he'd removed a fourth undetected spot but seemed very positive that he'd removed everything. I was over the moon and barely paid attention once he'd given me my travel clearance!

In a rush of excitement, Gem and I debated our itinerary. I was elated that things post-surgery had moved so quickly and I now had the freedom to introduce Gem to the immeasurable beauty of South Africa. Privately I had been a little more nervous than I admitted, there was a possibility that things may have not gone ahead so swiftly. But here we were, departure imminent! Mission accomplished.

My last two doctors' appointments were positive, the last even implying that I may be in the clear. Although the head histologist hadn't signed off on it yet everyone else had looked at it and the results had come back as benign! He would call me soon if anything changed but he honestly believed that I shouldn't be too worried anymore. That was the best news ever! Not only was I leaving on an amazing road trip but I had basically been given the all clear. Hello dream-life, here I come. I had made the right decision to ignore Dr Moneybags and follow my dreams. I was truly free in every sense of the word.

The next day we left before dawn heading for Kruger National Park. It was finally time for the real Africa; wild animals, dirt roads, scorching hot weather and spectacular views. We headed along the coast to Durban, enjoying beautiful hikes and even doing a cage-free dive with Black Tip Oceanic sharks! Clever baboons tried to break into our car and I'm convinced our smug little GPS took us on the world's bumpiest roads simply for its own amusement! We revelled in the glorious sun and stunning ocean scenes finally making it to Cape Town four weeks down the track. I relished not having heard from any doctors, the cancer once again fading into the past.

I welcomed in the New Year with good friends on the beach, champagne held high. I cast a wish that 2015 would be a year of change, promise and excitement; back to living my whirlwind life with no more cancer scares. I released all the stress of the year, eager to embrace the new unstoppable chapter of my life: because nothing could be as hard as a cancer scare at twenty-one.

Climbing Table Mountain signalled the finale of our trip together. Watching the sunset over the bay with Gemma is one of my most lasting and beautiful memories. We would have to leave soon but I was incredibly pumped about SCUBA diving every day for six months! Yes, let me repeat — every single day for nearly 182 days straight.

~ Broken Signals ~

It was Gem's last day and we were browsing around one of the big bustling markets with my dad. My youngest sister Amy was there too, having flown over recently to spend time with Dad. I was admiring the beautiful beadwork and quirky wood carvings when he missed a phone call. I dismissed it as a business call.

Later, getting back in the car, amid the chatter of happy shoppers, Dad interrupted suddenly.

"Jess, that message was from Dr Sunnies office – they sounded desperate to see you and asked us to come in as soon as we can."

My heart flopped over in my chest. Why where they desperate? They gave me the all clear so what could be wrong now? Did we just miss a check-up? Perhaps that's it. I'm cancer free – at least I'm supposed to be! I mentally slammed those thoughts shut just so I could function that day. I felt deeply uneasy but I refused to delve further. After a rough and sleepless night, I said a sad goodbye to Gemma the next morning. Somehow, I had to turn and face Dr Sunnies and his staff that afternoon.

My horrible nagging feeling followed me around all day. I dragged myself into the waiting room where Dad had already arrived. As I sank beside him, he turned to face me seriously.

"Dr Sunnies called me earlier. He didn't want to blindside us when we got inside." What was he talking about – how could I be blindsided? Why would we need to be prepared – this doesn't make any sense! *"The histology report has come back as melanoma."*

A shockwave went through me. Confusion crowded my mind.

"But they didn't call!"

My beautiful dream life instantly shattered into thousands of tiny pieces.

"They did try to call Jess, they tried and tried and for whatever reason they didn't get through, they have known for a month and they weren't able to get a hold of us."

My mind whirled in a vortex of confusion. Time slowed down, and it felt like I death-marched into that doctor's office.

Dr Sunnies apologised for giving me a false sense of hope. The head histologist was supposed to be the final person to sign-off on the report but he'd detected the presence of melanoma and then wanted it checked by other labs around the world before getting final confirmation. Despite having the right phone number, for some unknown reason they just could not get through to tell me. Sometimes I wonder if fate chose to give me those previous weeks with Gemma as a last gift of innocence.

Dr Sunnies wanted me on the chemotherapy eye-drops immediately and said that I'd need to be closely monitored. That caught my attention, *"So I can stay? I don't have to go home?"*

In all this bad news, I found the one thing I could be excited by.

"I'm not too sure; you need to see an oncologist and we'll decide from there."

This dulled my chances somewhat but I would hold onto that hope I always found! Dr Sunnies had also noticed a small mole on my lower lid. Even I wasn't sure if it was new or maybe it had been there for years. He wouldn't take any chances and booked another surgery for two days' time.

We booked an appointment with the recommended oncologist and I tried to organise my thoughts. I was convinced that if I was adamant with the doctors that I did not want to leave, I could still be on the beaches of Sodwana in a month.

I would be extra careful of course, using lots of sun protection and diligently returning to Johannesburg for monthly check-ups. It could all work out with good communication and planning. A bit of inconvenience, but I could work past that and finally become a SCUBA instructor.

~ Shattered Dreams ~

Dad, Ash and Amy came to the hospital with me for my next surgery. They munched on chocolate croissants while I lay in bed fasting and grumpy; all I wanted was a coffee and a pastry; was that too much to ask?

Amy was flying home that day so we had to say goodbye before I went into theatre. The surgery was a little more involved this time, Dr Sunnies took a wedge out of my eyelid and then stitched it back together. He undertook a proper scope of my eye to ensure it was clear. He seemed confident and had anticipated this surgery to be the least painful of all of them.

However post-surgery something felt off. Dad had taken Amy to the airport so it was just Ash with me. My eye kept continually watering and she was carefully wiping away the tears as they formed. As the drugs wore off though she laughed how fast my attitude changed to, *'Don't worry, it's just my eyes watering – it's fine.'* I was back to normal, sassy Jess!

In my recovery at home, my eye became really irritated like something was scratching it, I assumed it was the stitches. The awful discomfort made me snappy and then I started running a fever. Dad called Dr Sunnies who was surprised at my condition. With some extra painkillers, we made it through to the appointment four days after surgery. By then I wanted answers!

Within seconds of reviewing my eye, Dr Sunnies started chuckling. Huh? Was I overreacting? Being dramatic?

He carefully plucked something out of my eye and my goodness, the relief was instant and intense. When they had stitched my eyelid back together, a tiny eyelash had been pointing backwards – oh the irony of such a tiny thing causing so much pain.

Relief flushed over me when he told me the mole had come back as benign, and that I might not have to rush home to Australia after all. My smile was immense as I envisioned running along the Sodwana sand in my wetsuit ready for a dive at dawn. Dr Sunnies tried to temper my joy a little, advising me to wait until I got the all clear from the oncologist before making plans. I couldn't help it. I was bouncing back to my old self — no more lying around in a dark room for me; cramming in dinners, garden parties and BBQs before the next appointment. I even slept well for the first time in ages.

When the morning rolled around for my oncologist appointment, in a weird way I was feeling pumped; I was sure it was the day to put it all to rest and move forward. Dad and Ash were there with me as I met the oncologist, Dr Realist, who asked me about my diagnosis and the referral from Dr Sunnies.

As he read through the histology report, the minutes ticked by loudly and I watched his brow deepen as he jotted down notes. My palms suddenly felt clammy and I began to fidget, this wasn't going the way of the quick consultation I'd imagined. Dad put his arm around me, which only heightened my doubt.

Finally, he sighed, *"I think it best you go back to Australia. They are far beyond us in melanoma research and your medical expenses will be covered by the government there."*

I protested immediately in typical stubborn Jess style. *"No, I don't want to go back! Can't we manage it from here until July? Unless it becomes absolutely necessary for me to go home it's not something I intend on doing."*

He became blunt.

"Jess, I don't think you understand; melanoma kills. It is one of the nastiest and most aggressive cancers we encounter and it is not something to play games with."

I was suitably shocked into submission as he continued. *"You will need to undergo a P.E.T scan, blood tests and liver scans, which will cost upwards of R50,000 (AUD$5000). In Australia, they'll do these for free and when you're better you can come back."*

I wanted desperately to keep protesting but somewhere a voice said not to be stupid enough to risk my precious life for a holiday.

Dr Realist also checked my glands, showing me how to watch for any changes. *"You are the only one that knows how you're feeling. Look for any changes, discolouration of moles, swollen glands. It's up to you to monitor your health and let your doctor in Australia know immediately if you detect any changes."*

Suddenly I felt like I was on active duty, looking for any nasty potential cells that could attack at any moment. I avoid doctors at the best of times and now I was being told that I needed to tell them if I got a cold! It seemed like overkill. But at the first sign of swollen glands, I did go into panic mode. Has it spread? Can they even tell? What if I cough and they just think it's a normal cough and then months later I discover it's spread to my lungs and there is nothing they can do?' It might sound irrational but it's definitely something I thought about the first time I got the flu!

Following the doctor's bombshell, the three of us walked numbly down to the hospital café.

"How are you feeling?" Dad asked. I'm sure he knew the answer but perhaps understood that I needed to vent my frustration.

"I'm angry! I don't want to go home. I do not want this to control my life and if I go home—this beast of a thing wins!"

Dad wanted me to stay in South Africa but I couldn't let him throw away that kind of money on my medical costs. I knew I should consult Mum but I delayed the call for a few hours. I knew she'd tell me to come home but I wasn't ready to accept that was my only option. I wrestled with the corner I was backed into.

I kept holding onto the small hope that Dr Sunnies might tell me he can handle it, that he's confident it's all gone. I told Mum that I refused to come home unless I was really sick and I didn't feel sick at all.

Mum was prepared to pull out all the parental stops and asked to speak to Dad. *"Craig! She is not staying there – I want her home now – I want her to see the doctors here – this is a life or death thing – stop letting Jess put her life on the line – book her on a flight home immediately!"*

If there's one thing I've learnt from my cancer diagnosis, it's that parents of cancer patients feel the pain and grief just as much as their child fighting it. Parents are wired to save their children, protect them, throw themselves under a bus for them, and yet against this beast they can't fight it. There is an unspoken order to mortality but once you've been given this life-threatening diagnosis, your parents have to accept that they can't do anything to change it!

I returned the following day for Dr Sunnies to remove my stitches; I could barely see where I'd had the surgery. The only thing left was a cyst on my conjunctiva (the white part of my eye). I told him about the tests Dr Realist wanted done, the likely treatment and finally that he had recommended I go back to Australia.

Any hopes I'd had that Dr Sunnies would say it was manageable from his point of view were quickly dashed.

"That's what I've been thinking, Jess. You just can't risk it, go home, get checked, get over this bump in the road and then come back. The more research I do the more I realise that it's the only place for you to be and it would be foolish not to go back to Australia, they are miles ahead of us in melanoma research."

Now, I did understand his point; that the threat was very real – in theory. But to have all my hope and positivity from the start of that week ripped from underneath me, felt like a sledgehammer to my stomach. I simply could not equate that I was twenty-one, felt so fit and healthy and that my dreams, my volunteering, my diving, my whole life was being dictated to by some nasty invisible cells that had turned on me! I felt utterly stripped back and shattered to the core.

I wailed internally; I'm a good person, I've done everything right, so why is this happening to me? It was so unfair! Why couldn't it happen to some asshole who hits his wife, or a rapist or child molester? Does Karma not apply here?

I was so inflamed with injustice after the appointment that instead of going home, Dad took me to a bar near the hospital. Not necessarily to talk, but to let me rant and slam drinks down on the table in repeated outbursts of aggravation and disappointment at leaving South Africa.

I couldn't have known at that point, that melanoma is a constant battle, not something that can just disappear. You don't get rid of it with a bout of antibiotics or even in my case, surgery. It's there with you for years to come, waiting silently to potentially rear its nasty butthead when you're not looking! The bastard thing.

I tried to lift my spirits and packed as much as I could into the time I had left; markets, shopping and dining with family and friends. On my last night, I ate my weight in pork spare ribs from the finest family feast fit for a king! There were so many tears and hugs, I felt like I had just arrived and none of us were ready for this abrupt goodbye.

I still couldn't fathom that I felt so well yet was somehow sick enough to be sent home. It seemed like a faraway idea and it wasn't until we were leaving that night that it hit me that this might be the last time I see these people, my family. I hugged my grandpa and thought, 'cancer kills, I might not make it through another year, it might be my last goodbye.' I just wasn't ready for that. I couldn't keep myself together anymore and I sobbed my eyes out.

I was mentally and physically drained. I was on thin-ice, this fucking illness may cut my life short and there was nothing I could do to stop it. I still whinged at the universe, how dumb this situation was. I knew it was pointless but when options are severely limited you clutch at anything. I wished that a miracle would happen, that the doctors got it wrong, that they'd mixed the results up with someone else's, that I could stay and I'd be fine.

Once I'd played out that fantasy to its impossible conclusion, I accepted something. I knew going home meant we could sort this out, lay those manic thoughts of 'what if' to rest. The universe had made my bed and I had to lie in it. I finally accepted what was going on and decided I was going to fight this battle head-on and with all my might, no matter what.

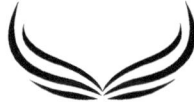

CHAPTER 3

THREE STRIKES

"There will always be rocks in the road ahead of us.
They will be stumbling blocks or stepping stones; it all
depends on how you use them."
— *Friedrich Nietzsche*

I would miss Johannesburg and its crazy manic appeal, it may not be beautiful but it holds a dear place in my heart and I hated leaving it behind.

A silver lining to my flight home was spontaneously meeting my cousin David while checking in. He was actually on the same flight to Australia as me. What luck – thank you, universe! I had seen David only a month prior while staying with his family in Port Elizabeth. Back then, it had been clear sailing for me so imagine his surprise to hear how quickly things had changed. We managed to sit next to each other on the plane and it made my reluctant trip home a thousand times easier.

We parted in Sydney for my connecting flight to Melbourne. Even though home was the last place I wanted to be, I couldn't deny how much I was looking forward to a big ol' Mumma bear hug!

Coming in to land, I felt overwhelmed and trapped by this disease once again. The one thing keeping me sane in that moment was the knowledge that my mum was the one person I could rely on to get the best doctors on my side. There was an irony to the way I had resisted her directions while away, but now they were a safety-net I relied on. When the announcement came to fasten our seatbelts for landing, I was so relieved the flight was over that I desperately wanted to crawl up in bed and bawl my eyes out (maybe punch a pillow or two as well).

I dragged my 36 kg of luggage around the airport, walking lopsidedly desperately looking for coffee! I must have looked ridiculous with bags hanging all over me but the soy mocha frappe was so worth it!

I was still irrationally annoyed though when Mum called to say she would be late picking me up due to an accident on the freeway. Then later she called to say meet her out the front of the airport! Not really appreciated by an emotionally jet-lagged girl with way too much luggage who should have forked out the $4 for a trolley. Once I eventually made it outside Mum saw me and raced around the car for the warm hug I'd been waiting for; I almost broke down right by the side of the road. I was tired and quiet on the long drive back to Mt. Eliza, a few mumbled replies to Mum's endless questions. It was fabulous to walk through the front door to a barrage of sibling hugs and chatter but I was desperate to hit my pillow and fall thankfully into the oblivion of sleep.

Mum wanted to start with a doctor we could rely on and the next day, I met her lovely GP, an exceptionally tall and thin man who towered over me like a beanpole. It can seem surreal meeting a new doctor for the first time and blurting out the sticky words of your cancer diagnosis. Dr Bean was amazing and immediately organised appointments for me at all the right hospitals. I would need a skin check the following week and he also organised the referral from Dr Sunnies.

Dr Bean was referring me to a classmate of his who had studied in South Africa but now practiced in the eastern suburbs of Melbourne. I called as soon as I left Dr Bean's office and they were able to squeeze me in for an appointment in ninety minutes. There's nothing like getting on with the job!

The referred doctor proved very interested in my case and the fact that I knew Dr Sunnies. It was the first time in eight years he had seen my type of cancer. He was sincere and said that he didn't feel he was the right doctor to see me through, but was happy to see how he could best help. I felt comfortable in his presence and mentally nicknamed him Dr Heart.

Between Dr Bean and Dr Heart and their referrals, not to mention lots of pestering phone calls their receptionists made on my behalf, I was in at the Victorian Eye and Ear Hospital the following Friday. I was also insanely grateful that Dr Heart gave me his long consultation non-gratis. A little different from good ol' Dr Moneybags. Anyone who has been through a similar diagnosis will know that even though our Medicare system is amazing, when you are seeing doctors four times a week it makes a large dent in your wallet.

After an interminably long wait for my first appointment at the Eye and Ear Hospital, it was a relief to finally be called in to meet the initial doctor. He read through my long case file and ran more tests. He then wanted to bring in his supervisor who was the leader in the field of Ophthalmic Oncology in Melbourne. I exhaled deeply with relief. I finally felt that I was in the right place, and my treatment would be in the hands of the most knowledgeable people, possibly in the world!

The next doctor entered. He was a tall white-haired gentleman with a kind, wise and wrinkled look. He wore an incredible wooden watch that I instantly noticed. I commented on it and he told me it was from South Africa; his son had purchased it for him. Our South African connection led to some comfortable chit-chat which certainly broke the ice. Dr Watch was also a brilliant and extremely straightforward man, thinking long and hard before sharing his view on my condition. He had moments of sounding overly direct and insensitive but I can honestly say on reflection that there is no other doctor that I would rather have been treated by. He looked through my file and was happy that the moles had been removed well with good margins. He explained that treatment from then on would just be local monitoring and a check-up every six weeks.

"We work in stages, first we aim to save the sight, if we can't do that we save the structure and finally we do whatever we can to save the life. Right now, you're in the first stage and by the looks of things that is where you will stay."

I was stunned. *"So we don't need to do any other tests? There is no other treatment I need?"*

"Nope that's it, you can just go back to living a normal life; you can go back to uni and work. Right now, we have it under control so putting your life on hold is pointless."

Man, was I angry and pissed off! I had been ready to fight this thing so I could go back to living life on my terms. Instead I flew all the way home to hear I was fine and I could go back to living my life! Except by then I had no money – I was stuck at home – and realistically I could have been back in South Africa living out my dream. This was too much! *"Well, can I travel if I'm fine?"* I needed to know.

He was reluctant. *"We would prefer you didn't but we can't stop you."*

From then on all I heard of the conversation was, 'as long as you don't miss an appointment with us you'll be fine.' I managed to thank the doctor and mentally stomp my way out.

I held my tongue until the privacy of the car. Mum had the pleasure of listening to me rant and rage all the way home in peak-hour traffic. I was so angry; this cancer thing felt like a joke! One minute it wrecks a path of destruction through my dreams and the next minute I'm told to just go back to uni! Huh? Thanks for that pointless wild goose chase. I felt dizzy with the quick turnaround from cancer to cure when in fact I had actually been 'cured' when I was in South Africa.

~ False Reprieve ~

I decided not to go back to uni for the next semester. I was so disappointed when the volunteering I'd planned as a Nutritionist in South Africa fell through, that I wasn't ready to face studying again yet. I was still too removed from my studies to concentrate. Plus, my classmates knew I was going to be away, I didn't fancy going back having to explain that I had a false alarm for cancer so here I am back early.

It was a confusing, unfulfilling time because surely no one gets off scot-free with a cancer diagnosis. I thought all this stress and dread can't have been for nothing. I felt a mixture of gratitude and resentment for all that I'd lost trying to get through it. Where did it leave me now? I decided to work and save up for a small trip to Bali to get my mind off all this bullshit. Mum tried to argue about the travel but I wasn't having a bar of it, I needed something exciting to look forward to so I didn't go stir-crazy. Mum knew that once my mind was made there was no turning back.

The rest of my family didn't understand my anger. I know I should have been relieved, and in many ways I was, but I also hated that my life had been tipped on its head and I didn't know which way was up.

Life quickly went back to mundane rituals scattered with doctors' appointments. The excitement of home and friends had worn off and I was on a comedown. In less than a month I was in a rut and felt brain-dead as I filled my days with waitressing at a café. I was looking forward to my exciting Bali trip but it was taking ages to arrive.

When April rolled around everything was looking pretty good from the doctors' point of view. Dr Watch decided on another surgery to remove a cyst that had been getting bigger on my eye. He didn't think it was anything to worry about but he wanted to be cautious. He wasn't too impressed that I was going overseas but as he said, "I can't stop you."

Two weeks before Bali, I was booked for surgery. I was becoming a seasoned professional when it came to eye surgery. I still hated fasting, especially as I was booked for the afternoon slot this time. My sister Britt came along for support and we listened to the anaesthetist explain the options of a local or general anaesthetic. Britt could see I was leaning towards the general and she thought the local was a way 'cooler' option so she dared me, promising to bring me Pellegrini's take-away if I did. She knows I can't turn down a dare, so I found myself answering 'local'. Later, I confessed that I had been dared and was actually really scared. She laughed good-naturedly and reassured me through every step as I counted backwards and fell under the spell of anaesthetic.

I felt myself waking up quite soon and unfortunately, this is where we found out I was metabolising the anaesthetic faster than normal and I could start to feel everything. Not to the fullest pain but I had to bite my tongue as Dr Watch finished up. I didn't relish ever repeating that experience but at least I only had to sit in recovery for a few minutes because of the local.

Mum and Britt were waiting for me with a massive serve of pasta – gnocchi — one of my favourite meals ever. That was my only reprieve for the next day or two as the pain set in and all I could do was recover in bed with painkillers (and another huge indulgence parcel from mum!).

After a few days of moaning I realised my old self was back again, with an added spring in my step because Bali was creeping up. I was so excited to get away and go hiking and diving. I started packing my bag as soon as I could get out of bed for long enough. Finally, a bit of freedom. A sense of normality which for me meant adventure! I was a bit uneasy about my money situation because I had taken time off work for the surgery, but I filed that away in my 'worry-about-that-another-day' mental compartment.

Into the beauty of Bali, I escaped! Letting the fear, the stress, the disappointment and the monotony of my life melt away. It was an incredible holiday where I relived my South African dreams by going scuba diving, hiking and embracing the freedom. I imagined my life was some version of exciting, even if I was only away for ten days. It was ten days of pure and juicy living.

Upon my return, I had the inevitable check-up with Dr Watch. I was in his office for all of ten minutes! He rechecked my eye, checked the surgery results and declared everything looked fantastic. He mentioned that I might have a freckle develop or other discolouration occur but I had nothing to worry about. He was happy to lengthen my reviews to every four months. This cancer thing was really starting to feel like a thing of the past.

However, I left the office feeling a bit tumultuous. On one hand it was fantastic that I was stepping away from this cancer world so quickly. I felt light, free and extremely lucky. On the other-hand though, I felt like the safety-net I had been cradled in over the last six months had been sliced open. I felt lost – free falling – trying to grab hold of what was happening but it was all so fluid. I felt alone and scared ... all of which no one else understood because to them I had been given good news. But layered within that, I'd lost all that had been consistent; all the support, all the knowledge that if anything were to go wrong I had a doctor's appointment just around the corner.

~ Wait For It ... ~

The knots in my stomach relaxed within a few days. No more long waits in boring hospitals with boring white walls, no more driving to and from hospital, no more being poked and prodded. This change was going to make it a lot easier to work and study.

I buried that little monster down deep as I refocused on my life going forward. I would start back at university soon and began to think about celebrating my birthday. If there is one thing I had learnt already thanks to my stint with cancer was that life is a blessing and we should celebrate everything within it, including turning 22!

Two weeks into my semester when I was putting on some mascara, I noticed a few small but extremely dark spots on my eye. I was overcome with panicked denial. I also found an unusual lump the size of a peppercorn on the inside of my lower eyelid. It felt hard but with a small amount of movement.

I was overwhelmed and confused trying to consider my next step. Dr Watch had advised me to expect discolouration on my eye, but something about these spots and that weird lump didn't sit right with me. That little monster wanted to burst out if its box but I wouldn't let it. I booked in to see my GP, Dr Bean instead. I didn't want to be a burden, to bother anyone, to cause everyone more stress and then be wrong about it.

Dr Bean knew a thing or two about melanoma. He took one look at the new spots on my eye, felt the new lump and was immediately on the phone to the Victorian Royal Eye and Ear Hospital, where

Dr Watch worked. My appointment with him was due soon anyway so I would have to maintain the status quo until then.

In the days leading up to it, I felt scattered. Just as I had managed to collect all the broken pieces of my life, some wicked demon had wretched them out of my hands, scattering them even further than last time. I honestly had no clue how to move forward, every time I tried to take a step away from this cancer journey, I was dragged back in by something bigger and scarier.

I tried to plan for every potential outcome I could think of. I both dreaded the appointment and wanted it at the same time. I was so reluctant to hear Dr Watch's opinion yet I sensed I'd have more peace once I heard his answers to all the scenarios I was imagining and I would soon have a real-life action plan.

My granny came with me to my next appointment and I realised everyone else in that waiting room was grandma's age. I must have looked like a good granddaughter accompanying her granny to her appointment. This was the first of many moments where I felt the isolation of my condition.

I'm convinced that waiting rooms would test the patience of a saint. I guess that's why they're called waiting rooms. I was irritated and confused when a new doctor I had never seen finally called me in two hours after the scheduled time. Two hours!

While we settled into the diagnostic room, Granny and I could hear the details of the conversation in the next room. A much older woman was being told her melanoma had progressed and the next step was to remove her eye. We heard about the process and the lady's tears. We heard how effective false eyes can look and I thought to myself she would still look pretty damn normal.

After introducing himself, I quickly cut in to ask the new doctor where Dr Watch was. I was more abrupt than usual but another lesson I've learned through cancer, is that it's a time when everything is out of my control so I crave consistency and try to obtain control over any areas I can.

He said Dr Watch was away on a five-week conference and holiday. Internally I was panicked, three-million questions flying through my mind about this man's experience and credentials. What will this doctor know? What if he gets it wrong? Can I trust what he says? Give me back Dr Watch.

I found a forced smile to cover my anxiety and began to explain my recent changes. He examined my eye and felt the lump in my eyelid. There was a light-hearted moment when I wanted to show him some past medical photos on my phone. I accidently swiped too far and he copped an eyeful when he saw a body transformation photo of me in nothing more than skimpy purple lingerie! A photo I didn't even want my Granny to see let alone a doctor I'd known for three seconds! I blushed, but soldiered on as though nothing had happened. Dr Blush tried to remain professional but after that over-share, eye contact was minimal and blushing at an all-time high! I like to think I added a little colour to his day. Purple to be specific.

Dr Blush concluded that the lump in my eyelid was just a blocked tear duct needing to be massaged every day. The new moles however looked very suspicious and I'd need to undergo another biopsy, he could fit me in quite soon. While I felt uneasy about having another doctor operate, I wasn't going to wait around for another month to see Dr Watch, so with very little hesitation I booked in for yet another surgery.

Mum was relieved when I told her about the lump and she brought home a few eye masks from work to help the massaging. This blocked tear duct diagnosis did not sit right with me, deep down I suspected there was something more to it, but I wanted so much for this to work so I still gave it a shot!

I began to mentally prepare for another surgery while also worrying about my Grandpa Eddie who had been admitted to hospital due to reduced lung capacity and severely low oxygen levels. Between the two of us my family were spending far more time in hospital than we thought possible!

I enjoyed a beautiful hospital visit with him one Sunday, an intimate time together. I so admired his resilience in the face of the pain I could see he was in. His arms where purple and bruised all over from the copious blood tests and drips that had been needed. It hit me how sick he was and how painful his experience was, both emotionally and physically. This would be the last time I would see my grandpa before he passed away. It's a day I now hold close to my heart.

Unfortunately, soon after that visit, I caught a nasty cough and chest infection. I was banned from visiting Grandpa again, both for his health and my own. My illness caused some infuriating miscommunication from the hospital, and my surgery had to be rescheduled. I was disappointed that this new date would now clash with a compulsory prac I was meant to do for one of my university subjects. I would have to drop the unit as neither obligation could be moved so my health would have to trump my study for the time being, another bump in the road.

Thankfully the surgery finally occurred under a local anaesthetic again, and as a devoted food lover, the sooner I eat after surgery, the better for everyone!

Dr Blush seemed a little concerned after the surgery. While he got most of the moles, he said my eye was very delicate due to all the surgeries I'd had and he had not been able to remove one of the moles because it was so close to the lump on the tear duct.

While he didn't articulate his concern, Mum and I could sense the undercurrent and conceded that perhaps the 'blocked tear duct' was a bigger worry than originally thought. While I had become a seasoned professional at recovering from these ocular surgeries, this recovery was much worse. I left the hospital high on pain medications and ready to eat, but when we went to our favourite restaurant nearby, I was overthrown with agony as soon as my lasagne arrived. I begged Mum to get more medications and take me home, while the staff thoughtfully bagged up my recovery meal for later! What followed was my longest recovery thus far, in bed with painkillers for days and then the nervous waiting and speculating before we'd get the results.

~ Fare Thee Well ~

Four days post-surgery, I felt well enough to go to a farewell brunch for a close friend before he left to study in Sweden. Due to my medications, I couldn't drive so a girlfriend picked me up. Mum had called me that morning to say Grandpa wasn't doing too well and to call past my grandparents' place as soon as I was finished brunch.

Instead of racing to my grandparents' house after brunch, I continued on with my friends for a cocktail (yes, I know shouldn't have while on medication) but I couldn't resist a little escape from the reality of what was happening in my life. I thought I still had time. I didn't understand the urgency. Mum called again, *"Where are you?"* Mum implored me to come over immediately. When I realised we had all been drinking and I couldn't get there quickly, panic set in. My brother raced to get me and then my youngest sister who was still at work.

Grandpa had passed away by the time we arrived.

I never got to say goodbye to him, to hug him one last time, to tell him I loved him. This was such a defining moment for me, because it was the first time I had lost someone so close to me that I could have said goodbye to but didn't. My brother sat in the room for hours with grandpa's body. I couldn't bear to be in there for more than a few minutes. Not because I am afraid of death or dead bodies, but because that cold frozen body was no longer my grandpa; his soul was at peace now and I found no solace in a dead man's body.

I believe in heaven, in a life after death and therefore our bodies are just our vessels on earth. In contrast, my brother doesn't believe this which gave grandpa's body far more importance. It was all that was left of our grandfather and he wanted to cherish the moments with him while he still could.

Later when everyone was asked to pick a flower from Grandpa's beloved garden I chose one of his enormous lemons because they were his pride and joy. This was the day I learned the fragility of life, that we can easily be there one day and gone the next. It was the day I promised myself to never miss out on an opportunity to say goodbye to a loved one again.

~ The Drastic Approach ~

With my surgery and my grandpa's passing I fell further and further behind in my studies. I managed to get extensions on all my impending assignments but I was also becoming overwhelmed with everything I had on my plate and all the uncertainty I was facing. It was a very intense period.

To my surprise, when results day arrived we were seen right away by Dr Watch. The first thing I asked was 'where's Dr Blush?' I was really struggling with the revolving door of doctors. As soon as I began to trust a doctor they were removed from my life. It's so important to have a level of consistency when everything else feels so out of your control! I had known Dr Watch would return but I was not expecting to never see Dr Blush again, he was no longer even at the hospital. (At least, hopefully I left him a memorable 'purple' moment to remember me by.)

Dr Watch didn't waste time and quickly confirmed my deepest fears. Every single mole that had been removed was malignant melanoma!

He avoided eye contact with me as he continued.

"We have a three-strike policy and this is your third strike."

The consultation room suddenly felt both bigger and darker, like it could swallow me up whole. Even with Mum by my side, I felt deeply alone. Dr Watch again felt the lump underneath my eye and without a second thought said, *"It's spreading and much faster than I expected."*

"So, it's not a blocked tear duct?" I said in a slow confused tone.

"No, it's a melanoma tumour," he said. *"We need to take a far more drastic approach this time."*

His voice held little emotion. To him it was just a fact, the next step forward. For me it was like I had started rolling down a mountainside. A nudge to begin with, but with each word, each statement, I was picking up speed and careening down the mountain face and spinning out of control.

Neither Mum nor I knew how to respond. We sat there slack-jawed, looking for some silver lining, waiting for him to reveal the way out of this mess. Dr Watch kept scribbling notes at his desk.

Finally Mum asked carefully, *"What do you mean by drastic?"*

"We're going to have to take the eye."

WHACK!

What?! WTF?!

The words slapped into my face. *Take the eye! What do you mean?*

He'd said it like it was supposed to be obvious. But my little ball of life as I knew it had finally hit the bottom of the mountain at full-pelt and burst open into an unrecognisable puddle of goo.

Numbness flooded my body. Robotically I reached out to take the three referrals he'd written. The first for a head/brain MRI, the second for a skin melanoma oncologist to which I questioned the need for.

"Well I'm an eye specialist, now that the melanoma is in the eyelid as well, it's spread to the skin and I need their input as to how to deal with this during the next surgery."

The last one was for a Youth Cancer Centre where Dr Watch said I would get emotional support and counselling for the next steps forward. I couldn't contain it anymore and I exploded.

"You can't just send me off to someone and hope they can counsel me into agreeing to let you take my eye!"

Dr Watch looked up in shock but in a very matter of fact tone replied, *"I know they can't but they will help you accept what's going on."*

I couldn't speak another word and left fuming. I'm sure the entire waiting room was staring as hurricane Jess tore through with angry and frustrated tears streaming down her face!

I wasn't angry at Dr Watch, or even the services he had offered; I was angry at the universe, at life, or more accurately — how my life was turning out. It didn't seem fair, there had to be another option, another way to deal with this that didn't end in me having a fucking glass eye!

It was an erratic few days. Besides my bombshell, the whole family was feeling the upheaval of losing Grandpa and preparing his funeral. I was just reacting to everything and running around following directions.

I tried to calm down and actually consider the possibility of having a glass eye. I would still be able to work, drive and study and surprisingly I would only be losing 10% of my vision. I could make the iris whatever colour I wanted – which for me would obviously be purple. I thought maybe, just maybe, it wouldn't stop me moving towards my goals and it won't be too bad. I decided to see a counsellor from the Youth Cancer Centre to help get some clarity to it all.

The funeral was emotionally traumatic on two fronts. I was saying goodbye to my beautiful grandfather and realising my regret at not seeing him more before he had passed. The other was seeing all my extended family and explaining where my treatment was heading; that I was going to have to lose my eye. I was emotionally drained at the end of the funeral; I had nothing left to give, barely able to complete a sentence.

I often grapple with whether I am grateful that Grandpa passed away before we knew about my eye or if I wish he had been there. I am grateful that he was no longer in pain, however he was the only other family member who had been in and out of hospital so much, so in some ways he would have been the only one that understood what I was going through and how to help me.

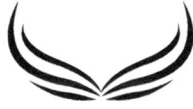

CHAPTER 4

THE RAW
HARD FACTS

"No one ever made a difference by being like everyone else."
— *P.T. Barnum*

Dad returned to help Mum and I navigate this mess. I was honestly terrified every step of the way, this was going to be my first ever MRI and I really didn't know what to expect. It was amazing to have Dad with me on those days because Mum couldn't keep taking days off work. He wasn't just there for the appointments, he kept me occupied and out of the house most days.

One day I remember in particular, it was the Tuesday before my follow-up with Dr Watch. Dad and I were sitting at one of my favourite cafés, the Seaford Beach Café, right on the waterfront overlooking the bay and the pier. It was overcast but still breathtaking, the tide was the furthest out I'd ever seen it. After brunch we bought takeaway coffees and wandered along the deserted beach. It was a beautifully serene walk, the calm before the storm. After a while Dad suggested we sit at one of the benches up on the embankment, I thought he was just tired of walking but when we sat down the mood shifted.

"I spoke to Dr Watch on the phone yesterday."

I was puzzled by this news but looked at him expectantly. My dad who is normally a straightforward, charismatic man was gazing downwards and shuffling his foot in the dirt. He was silent for a full minute as he gathered his words. I could feel his tension and my knuckles whitened as they wrapped themselves tighter around the bench.

"Dr Watch said he's going to have to remove your eye," he paused. *"I just don't want you to be blindsided on Friday."*

My hands instantly relaxed as I let out the massive breath I'd been holding. *"Dad, Dr Watch told Mum and I that last time we saw him ..."*

"Yes, but he didn't tell you everything."

Talk about a confusing statement. Isn't it simple, remove the eye and the tumour in the eyelid and then we're right as rain? I'd have a fabulous purple eye in no time.

"Jess he isn't just taking the eye, he has to take the eyelids as well ... and close the socket for good!"

My jaw dropped. Blood drained. Time stopped. Dread sprinted into my soul.

My mind exploded with a myriad of distorted horrifying images.

I would look like some patchwork doll, an eerie character like Sally from the movie, *The Nightmare Before Christmas*.

Tears streamed down my face uncontrollably as I realised these fucked-up, gruesome images would be *my reality*!

I was silent for a long time, literally lost for words. There were none to describe this nightmare. The horror that gripped my heart and mind.

I just kept seeing images flash by. I was falling down a black hole, without light or ending. The anger, the fear, the devastation boiled.

The world blurred, as I yelled.

"NO! FUCK that! Absolutely not! I am not parading around the streets looking like some freak show on display for the world to see! I'm not a circus act! How the fuck could he think this is even an option! He is a fucking moron if he thinks he can just con me into agreeing to this absurd surgery! I can't! NO way in hell is this happening! I would rather die than

let him do this."

Now I don't usually swear, but I had saved them all up to let out this rage inside me. It was a furious and frenzied storm. I vaguely thought how it now made sense why Dad chosen a relatively secluded spot to tell me. He just let me go on and on and on in writhing circles until I had nothing left to say and I felt empty inside. I finally slumped over; my body couldn't hold the weight of this burden.

~ The Search ~

Later, once I had gained some ability to function again, Dad acknowledged that he agreed with me.

"There is no way they're taking your eye. It's absurd! I've been up all night looking at other options and I have found a treatment that will work. It's called Keytruda and although it's very new, it seems to have fantastic results with melanoma."

I confess my face lit up at his words. We started planning our counterattack, we would research and present it at the next appointment with the skin specialist coming up.

With my parents by my side, I felt armed for battle as we strode into the appointment that Friday, all our credible research waiting to be fired like bullets of brilliance. This new hospital, Peter MacCallum Cancer Centre was massive, there were countless corridors and people heading in all directions. The long wait was exhausting considering we were so on edge, feet tapping, backs straight, ready to pounce as soon as they said my name!

Eventually a new doctor, led us to our consulting room. He was a Skin Melanoma Oncologist who specialised in surgery; he looked more like a mad professor than a doctor and was a very abrupt man. Between his questions, his instructions and his fancy charts, I felt like I couldn't get a word in. Dr Chart deftly examined my eye and the skin on my torso. *"You don't have melanoma type skin, but it's definitely a melanoma tumour."* As if that was a fact that should make me feel better.

Finally, there was a pause in his talk and I took that moment to pounce.

"Look, Dr Watch wants to do this ridiculous surgery and I am not going

through with it! I will not look like a freak for the rest of my life just because he deems it necessary."

Dr Chart replied firmly, he agreed with Dr Watch, *"This surgery is the best option, we need to take margins, and this is the only way to do so."*

I had reached my tipping point.

"You are not taking my eye and leaving me with some patchwork job! I refuse to look like some freak and I will not be going through with this surgery. There has to be another option, a different surgery that is not going to destroy my face! What about Keytruda? I've read a lot about the successes it's had." I was breathless with emphasis.

Dr Chart looked a bit taken aback, and reiterated that he believed my only option was surgery, however he would bring in two other specialists next week, one being a plastic surgeon, the other who would talk to me about Keytruda and other treatment options. Despite feeling extremely annoyed that he couldn't give me an answer on the spot – as though I was in the too hard basket – I felt confident that someone else on my case would help me.

Following this onerous appointment came some respite in the form of a beautiful nurse who spent a long time talking with me. Or rather just listening and handing me tissues and consoling me through the emotional rollercoaster I was on. From tears, to anger, to laughter and all over again, she understood that I was grieving. Not just the obvious distress about losing my eye, I was grieving the loss of the life I had envisioned for myself.

My future, my career, the love and future children of my own that looking different might take away from me. She really listened, like my voice mattered, reinforcing that all I was holding onto was valid, that I wasn't overreacting and I needed that. I needed to feel like I was normal even as normality was quickly fading. I needed to feel heard because even though she didn't have a solution, it was so comforting to know someone was listening. I needed to feel the attention was on me as a person, not on my diagnosis, not on my patient number but me; Jess, a living breathing human being with opinions and fears that were being tossed around. This nurse sat with us for hours, talking everything through. I never felt like she had somewhere else to be or like I was wasting her time. She helped me find my voice; to advocate for myself against the tide against me. She was an angel in one of my darkest moments; she was and still is my Nurse Angel.

~ Let's Hear It ~

We still had the appointment with Dr Watch to get through that day. In the madhouse of a waiting room, Mum had to sit alone while Dad and I sat hunched together over a notebook putting numbers down on paper, trying to work out what risks were worth taking. Losing my eye was a last resort and I planned on exhausting every other option before we went down that route.

I was really irritated. One of Dr Watch's interns had just tried to have a consultation with me that proved disastrous. When her opening gambit was the assumption I would comply with the surgery, I lost it! How dare she make such casual statements about my life and my decisions. I practically yelled at her that I was looking into other options and I would only discuss this with Dr Watch. She left in a flurry with tears in her eyes.

I was left both embarrassed and furious, trying to avoid eye contact with the watchful waiting room audience. Dr Watch called us in, he had four interns with him in the room, including the woman I'd railed at.

Dr Watch was always a commanding presence, but that day he really meant business, and he got straight to it.

Dr Watch: *"I hope you don't mind, I have brought these doctors in training to observe. I understand you spoke to Dr Chart this morning?"*

Me: *"Yes but ..."*

Dr Watch: *"And I see you went for the MRI this week. It shows that there is a problem area and it's still localised."*

Me: *"Yep, Dr Chart has also organised a PET scan, CT and chest X-ray for this coming Wednesday and I will be seeing him next Friday for a follow up appointment where he will present all our treatment options."*

I was proud to stand my ground reminding him that I will not be losing my eye under any circumstance.

Dr Watch: *"OK good. We have seen and removed one lesion and we've* seen multiple reoccurrences. If we treat it locally, 89% of people will not have a reoccurrence. Jessica, this is different, we have had 3 strikes against your eye, and the eye is a delicate organ. When we realise that there is a reoccurring problem and the eye is becoming unstable, we need to take something out and we need to work out how big that has to be. My view is that we have to be aggressive with our surgery, if we don't it will just keep reoccurring locally and become increasingly difficult to deal with. It can also spread. Melanoma unfortunately is a condition that many young people can get and a condition that people can succumb to. We should be surgically aggressive."

Me: "What about radiation?"

Dr Watch: "Radiation on the front of the eye is not viable because it is not contained. It would also damage the skin and the bone if we go down that line. If surgery needed to be done later it would be compromised due to blood supply being affected, making the surgery far more difficult."

Dad: "And Keytruda?"

Dr Watch: "They are good drugs, but we do not use them in the primary setting because surgery is much better at controlling it early."

Dad: "I understand what you're saying, especially if you're sixty-years-old but at twenty-two when you have your whole life ahead of you — it seems rather harsh to lose your eye."

Dr Watch: "The decisions are even more important. In older people we make judgement on treatments and side effects. But I know that if we don't solve this problem Jess is not likely to be here in five years. Your best survival chance is with surgery. No surgery, death will be certain."

I felt backhanded across the face with an encyclopaedia. I didn't realise this was life or death! I didn't realise playing with treatments was also playing with my life and my future.

My heart sank deep into my stomach as I tried to grasp at the two realities I wanted; to stay alive and to look normal. However, they were on the other ends of the spectrum, choosing one meant losing the other. Tears poured down my face as I realised every option was being snatched away and all that was left was death or being socially ostracised.

I distantly heard Dad ask something further.

Dr Watch: "She would end up with a fungating tumour in the current location and it would more than likely spread. The problem with that is that the local treatment will become more difficult."

Dad: "Can you explain the surgery?"

Dr Watch: "The operation is to remove the contents of the organ, we would leave the eyelid skin, up to, but not including the eyelashes. You'll lose the muscle and the fatty tissue around it."

Dad: "If there is no muscle, Jess will have a prosthesis that can't move?"

Dr Watch: "We will join the skin together, the skin then sits in the hollow that is left there, and yes, it is unusual but it does enable you to wear a silicon prosthesis that sits in the socket and looks very realistic, it just will not move. Trying to rebuild this is virtually impossible."

Me: "So, then the eyelid won't move, it won't blink?"

I was dumbfounded, trying to wrap my head around this weird concept.

Dad: "No they will be closing it over. Permanently."

Me: "Then how does the prosthesis work?"

Dr Watch: "It sits externally."

Me: "It would look ridiculous!"

He did not seem impressed with my response and view on the matter.

Dr Watch: "It looks like a prosthesis that can be either mounted on thin glasses or on magnetic implants."

Dad: "So when you take the glasses off, there is just a blank behind that?"

Dad's choice of words was blunt but at this point none of us could understand exactly what was going on, what my future looked like. We were desperate to understand the ongoing impacts of such a drastic surgery and couldn't afford to sugar-coat our terminology.

Dr Watch: "There is a hollow."

Me: "I don't want that. I don't want that at all!"

Dad: "So this is harsh. This is really harsh."

Dr Watch: "None of us want any of this, the reality is we've been trying to avoid it, but we are out of options."

Me: "Can't you just maintain these muscles and put a prosthesis there? This just sounds horrific to me, I mean I'm 22."

I was sobbing – still clutching that there must be another option he wasn't telling me.

Dr Watch: *"The reason I am telling you all this is because of that very reason, you are 22, and the alternative is not as good as this. This offers you a pathway, nothing else does. We don't have a magic drug, ray or local surgery that can help us out at this point."*

Dad: *"So you don't see any other option?"*

Dr Watch: *"My role is to advocate what is the best option, and in my opinion, this is the only pathway to stop this spreading. I want you to talk to the radiation oncologist, the medical oncologist. We don't treat primary lesions with anything other than surgery. We need you to go through this process, get the scans, talk to the doctors and then get back in contact with me."*

Dad: *"To what? To say this is what we've decided? You say it like there's other options."*

Dr Watch: *"This is a decision that you three need to make, having talked to all the relevant professionals."*

Me: *"Are there any other options looks-wise?"*

I wasn't paying attention to what was going on around me, I was fixated, there had to be some alternative, some way to save my life and not look different to everyone else in the world.

Dad: *"Do you have any photos we can see? The photos online don't look particularly good. We want to know what it will look like without the eye there."*

Me: *"No I don't care about that, I want to know what other options I have for prosthesis false eyes, I don't want something that doesn't move!"*

Dad: *"There isn't, that's what they're saying."*

Me: *"Well then what's the point? It's just a plastic thing. I don't even need glasses!"*

Dad: *"There is no glass eye Jess, there are no eyelids. The reality is you need to know what it looks like without the prosthetic."*

Dr Watch: *"We can also drill a metal peg into the eye socket. The silicon can sit on the pegs. It will look a little bit unusual, and the whole point of the glasses is two-fold: it's a mounting point, and less surgery you don't need. Glasses are a visual focus, it takes away from the focus on the eye. You can tell, there is no way of getting away from that because it will not be moving. There is no way of making it move and movement is one of the things that can make a prosthetic eye look normal."*

Dad: *"It's just a dummy eye sitting on top of your skin."*

Me: *"I don't want it! I don't want to look weird."*

Dr Watch: *"I have also spoken to you about seeing the counsellors."*

Me: *"I don't need to be counselled through this!"* I spat back at him through the tears, I was furious, I felt manipulated, like he was panning me off to some other person to force me to make the decision he wanted me to.

Dr Watch: *"No, no, no it's not about that. You've got no experience in what it is to make tough decisions. What you are expressing to me quite clearly is that this is an undesirable outcome. But the alternative outcome is something you need to consider. We need you to understand risk."*

Me: *"Well I'd rather take the risk."*

Dr Watch: *"This is not a 10% risk, if we don't do anything there is 100% risk of dying. I want someone to teach you about decision-making. This is a decision-making thing where there is no good choice. How do you make a decision to go left or right when neither of them are decisions you want to choose? My role is not to help you make the decisions. I am here to give you the options."*

Dad: *"But there are no other options, that's what you keep telling us."*

Dr Watch: *"You keep saying she's 22 which is even more reason to make the decision that's going to give her a long-term chance. I'm not saying you can't make a decision Jessica but none of us have the firsthand experience in making difficult, personal choices. And we will support you with whatever decision you make, we will help you carry it out, even if that wasn't our advice."*

Me: *"It doesn't make any sense as to why all the eye parts need to go. Why can't you just rebuild it?"*

Dr Watch: *"On a technical level we cannot rebuild muscle and fat."*

Dad: *"All we can see [online] is people who have scars all the way down their faces, I mean what do you do with that, walk around with a patch?"*

Dr Watch: *"Well that's what some people do, I have one patient who has long hair and she hangs it over the eye, we tend not to take photos for personal reasons. We can also send you to the prosthetics person. If that's the way you want to go I'd suggest it's something you do before the surgery, this is not the way everyone decides to go."*

Dad: *"Well its better than waking up with a surprise after the surgery.*

We would like to have a good idea of what to expect before it happens."

Dr Watch: *"Like most of these significant operations, the anticipations are the most difficult part. It looks unusual, but most people after a while readily accept the way they look. We need to try and cure this cancer."*

Dad: *"The best way to make this easier is to know what it's going to look like, is it a big scar down her face or a small line?"*

It felt like I wasn't in the room, my questions, my stance was falling on deaf ears. And maybe for good reason, I was highly emotional; I wasn't grasping or accepting what was going on. I felt like a child who had no control over what was going on.

Me: *"Either way it's awful."*

Dad: *"One is worse than the other."*

Me: *"No it's not, it's all horrific, I will look like a circus freak."*

Dr Watch: *"It will look as if you had closed your eye and pushed it back in, it is a smooth cupped hollow. This is a lid-sparing exenteration and it will be a smooth transition, it will look a bit like your armpit. You are going to lose the eye no matter what we do."*

I sat in shock, an armpit on my face!

Me: *"I don't want to walk around looking different. It's just not fair."* I said helplessly. I could finally see there were no other options, but I still didn't want this one.

Dr Watch: *"I'm not saying it's an easy decision, it's not a decision any of us want to have to make."*

Me: *"This is just going to be so different and my career aim of being a dietitian is about seeing people and dealing with people, and if I look so different who is going to want to see that."*

My thoughts spiralled downwards; I would never be socially accepted. I would be unloved, unwanted, undesired like the lepers I had read about in the Bible when I was younger. I knew how society worked, that different is not accepted, that I would be stared at, ridiculed, ostracised. Who would want to be friends with me when they found out I would have an armpit where my eye was?

Dad: *"She's worried about finding a partner, about her career, about all the things that every young adult wants."*

Dr Watch: *"People do have to make decisions and are generally not good at making them, especially when we are in a lose-lose situation."*

Me: *"There is no other option. There just isn't. I am not making a decision, I am backed in a corner."* I felt pressured to make the life-saving decision.

Dr Watch: *"We can look at it and say that yes treatments and drugs are always improving but you are making a decision today, not in the future."*

Me: *"And there is no other way to make it look more natural?"*

Dr Watch: *"Essentially no. There are people who have tough decisions to make, there are children and young adults who do not survive cancer. A good decision is one that you decide on and live by."*

Me: *"What about sport?"*

Dr Watch: *"You can play sport, you can drive a car, your experience will be a bit different because you'll have one eye."*

At least that part of my life wouldn't be taken away.

Dr Watch: *"I'm going to keep moving, and you need to get moving because this is about decision-making."*

My eyes darted to my parents, begging for them to step in, hoping that they could turn this nightmare around. They looked as defeated as I did. It felt like I'd been in the ring with my doctor for twelve rounds dodging, punching, fighting back, but his jabs hit harder than mine, he'd worn me down and I broke. Tears of pure fear flowed through me. I had nothing more I could give, nothing more I could do. I felt like the cancer had won. Cancer had finally started impacting my life and there was nothing I could do. I knew that while the people around me could support me, for this journey I was flying solo. I had to make the decisions. I was the only one in this fight; everyone else was just giving their advice from the sidelines.

Mum told me later that it was one of the toughest moments in her life, she wanted so desperately to save me, to fix it all but there was nothing she could do or say to change it, so she just sat there and cried with me.

Dr Watch left the room, he didn't rush us out and we just sat there in doomed silence.

Eventually I said through sobs, *"I don't know if I can do the surgery. I don't want to be different. Life is going to be so different. I don't want that. I don't care if it ends in my death."*

I didn't see the implications of the words at the time, I didn't realise it would hurt Mum so much. She howled at the thought of me not being around, but I was just saying what I was thinking at the time.

"*Jess you have to. I need you here.*" Mum begged.

Dad took a more direct approach, "*Well you heard what he said, if you don't have the surgery you'll have a festering thing coming out of your face and you don't think more people will be staring at that?!*"

I was spent. I didn't talk for hours. I sat on my bed, staring blankly at my bedroom wall for about 24 hours straight. I just let myself sit in the mess of it all. I gave myself permission to feel, think and experience everything at full force, no barriers. I could laugh, I could cry, I could scream, I could punch pillows.

Initially there was a lot of anger, but once I let that out, I felt empty and ready for contemplation.

For the first time in months I was in an almost peaceful space, where I had all the facts. I contemplated life and death and all things in between. I had been so blessed to have such a full life at the age of 22. I had loved, I had travelled, been to the depths of the ocean and jumped out of a plane. I had laughed, chased dreams, and learned so many beautiful lessons.

I realised right then that if I were to die tomorrow I would have no regrets, and while my bucket-list was still long, I had been bold enough to take every opportunity that had come my way and knowing that was truly satisfying.

It was a surreal paradox how one solitary thought helped me come to terms with my mortality. Yet it also made it abundantly clear how beautiful my life was that I was willing to do whatever it would take to have more years on Earth living this amazing blessing we call life.

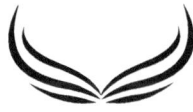

CHAPTER 5

THE DECISION THAT WOULD CHANGE MY LIFE FOREVER

"Life is ten percent what you experience and ninety percent how you respond to it."
— *Dorothy M. Neddermeyer*

I had made my decision.

This triggered another huge moral question. How would I come to terms with the surgery and the long-lasting effects it would have on my life? I ruminated for a long time asking myself who I was underneath the layers and what I would make out of this situation.

I could choose to be Jess, the 22-year-old freak, the poor girl who lost her eye and felt sorry for herself, who locked herself away in her room, who found a way to work from home so she would not have to interact with the outside world. The girl who was unloved, unaccepted, unwanted, a burden to her friends and family. I could see her clearly, sitting in her dark bedroom, with the blaring light of her laptop illuminating her face; full of fear and hatred. Her life was unfair. I couldn't stop the tears rolling down my face, it felt so real, I felt sorry for her. That girl on the bed looked like me but I felt something shift within me and knew it wasn't. This girl had lost her love of life, her passion, her shine. She had let the cancer win: she may well still be here but she was no longer living.

I knew who I wanted to be.

I could be powerfully positive Jess, a young woman full of confidence, who embraced life every day, who made the most of the hand she had been dealt. A woman who loved herself so fully, so wholeheartedly it was beautiful. She was beautiful. She didn't care what anyone else thought of her, she was strong and happy. She wore her scar with pride because she had chosen life over vanity.

She had her family and her friends supporting her, she was not alone. I saw her with the biggest smile on her face, her hands were on her hips in a power stance, she was surrounded by bright beautiful light and I could see her passion for life radiating from her. She was amazing and I was so proud of her, I wanted to *become* her.

None of us are guaranteed tomorrow but I was being offered a second chance at life with this surgery. If I chose to live a life as 'poor Jess' it was an insult to anyone who had died too young, because I knew that they would have chosen to lose an eye to save their life.

I had to honour myself, my family, but mostly I had to honour anyone that had passed away too soon. I made my choice in honour of them, because very few people get an opportunity to choose. It was an incredible moment realising I could become that powerfully positive Jess. So I asked myself the single most important question, *'How do I do that?'*

I wanted to embrace and own my actions, own my situation, be comfortable with looking different; be proud! I didn't want to hide behind some doll's face, pretending to be the same as everyone else, trying to fit in.

Elements of this ideal really challenged me and I had to break it down to my moral core. For so long I had believed that I would rather be recognised for who I was rather than for how I looked. I used to say openly that I would rather be recognised for being smart, funny, helpful, kind, loving or healthy than for the physical appearance I had no contribution into building.

I wanted to be recognised for the beautiful person I had created, not my genetic makeup. And now the universe was goading me as if to say, 'You're the one who said looks don't matter to you, prove it! Keep living, loving and learning despite all of this. It will make you stronger!' The journey would push me to breaking point and test my very foundations but if I couldn't hold onto my beliefs in the tough times, I realised I had never truly believed them.

With those fundamentals in place and the realisation that people were going to look and stare no matter what, I decided to be different, to own it; I wanted to wear an eyepatch! Not some plain black boring pirate-style one, I wanted colour, diamantes and glitter, a statement piece, my own unique accessory. I was going to make it part of my style and have fun with it.

I would have to exude confidence to pull it off and love the new me. I knew it wouldn't be easy in the beginning, that there would be days where I would want to hide away. I would have to fake it to make it. I looked for role models, people who had faced adversity but surmounted it with apparent ease.

I thought back to a time when I felt confident, really confident. I was at a university ball in an elegant black gown, and I started analysing that confidence. I walked with ease, almost as if I was gliding, my shoulders back, my head held high. My smile was so bright as I thought what an amazing night it was; that I was blessed to be there. I felt beautiful, strong and fun, with so much to offer the world. I knew that night could be my reference for confidence when it was lacking. I needed to do, think, say, and believe those things about me and I would feel more confident.

~ You Win Some, You Lose Some ~

With the decision to wear an eyepatch using confidence and self-love as the key, everything else became easier. It was Friday that I received the news about losing my eye and by Sunday I had become the eyepatch expert. I already knew where to find them and had a huge collection sitting in my checkout basket on the internet.

I was ready to tell my closest friends and family my plan and while I was still terrified of the surgery, I felt a flicker of excitement that I had taken this challenge in my stride. I felt calm and in control again.

Telling my loved ones individually and in person was really important. Even though I still needed their support, I wanted them to see that I was OK with my decision, that I knew the difficulty ahead but I had developed some incredible tools for how I would not let this define me, even how I could use it to become the person I wanted to be.

It wasn't easy, the conversations were all so different, some people were in support rallying behind me, some were in tears crying beside me and others found this news too much of a burden to bear. It either made my relationship with them stronger, or it broke down all together. As I comprehended the depths of my decision and my new outlook, I needed full support, needed my loved ones, needed my friends to help carry the weight of this burden, even carry me at times too.

I'm not going to lie and say that it was all sunshine, I lost some of my longest standing friends through this time and it was awful. I look back now and think it was a blessing because whether it had been this circumstance, or another, there always would have been something too hard to deal with and I would have lost them then. It taught me who my true friends were.

I had to reconcile that this decision was both permanent and visual. There was no way of tiptoeing around treatment and dealing with this quietly. I still lived in the area I grew up in, regularly bumping into all sorts of people that knew me. Anticipating that my news would spread fast, I wanted to be on the front foot, dispensing any gossip or false assumptions.

After sharing the news with those closest to me I decided to make a massive post on social media to address everything directly.

JVZ

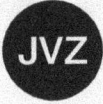

Jessica Van Zeil
8 September 2015

•••

"This week I have had to face the hardest decisions of my life. As most of you know I have been battling with Melanoma spots on my left eye for a few years now. To date I have had four operations and every time the spots keep coming back and grow faster and more aggressively. The spots are Melanoma cancer spots.

Three months ago, I developed a small lump on my bottom eyelid which has grown rapidly and unfortunately has now been confirmed as a Melanoma tumour.

I have been dealing with 2 different professors, one at the Peter Mac Cancer (Dr Chart) hospital and the other one at the Royal Eye and Ear Hospital (Dr Watch) in Melbourne. My family and I have had extensive meetings with both of them recently and unfortunately the only real and viable solution to this is pretty shitty to say the least.

Basically, this is a very aggressive form of cancer that does not respond to chemo or radiation very well, and if it is left untreated will lead to my death in less than 5 years.

The only option of surviving this cancer is the full removal of my eye, with no option of a glass eye. There is no other option. The decision comes down to a decision to live, to have life and to be able to live a cancer-free life going forward.

I have come to terms with what is going to happen, so please don't be scared to talk to me about it or avoid me when you see me.

As you can imagine this has been incredibly hard and emotional to process for me. But being the person that I am, I am going to face this head on and make the most of my life and the new me, just as I have always done. Rather than try and hide, I have decided that I am going to be proud of it and I am going to wear bold, bright, funky and glittery eyepatches. After all, I am a cancer survivor!

My sister Britt, really wanted to help in some way, and she enthusiastically set up a fundraising page for me called Eye Won. The momentum she created helped to support me in important practical ways. Not just funding eyepatches which are surprisingly expensive items but also for prescribed glasses, depth perception rehabilitation, medications, counselling, ongoing medical consultations not to mention the time lost from being unable to work. She also added some much needed humour to my life and to this day we still 'search' for my missing eye. We send photos to each other whenever we 'find' my eye; on billboards, handbags and even those googly eyes at craft stores.

Britt gave this project such fun, positive energy and it was humbling to see its amazing results and how it has helped me in unexpected ways. Seeing myself as winning, rising above the odds and not falling victim to this disease. We enjoyed some truly memorable time together in Sydney thanks to the sponsorship Britt generated.

~ Dr Energiser ~

Meanwhile, I had been getting back to business with Dr Chart. While I was still open to hearing from the other specialists, I was now prepared to move forward with the life-saving operation.

The situation was still complicated because while Mum backed me in this decision, Dad had still not accepted the surgery. He continued to research Keytruda, speak to other specialists and calling on friends in the medical field. Looking back, I can see that he was trying to protect his daughter from cancer. However, at the time this was causing havoc in our relationship, as Dad clung to hope of a miracle and I had moved on.

Dr Chart was forthright when we next sat down together. He explained a large group of melanoma experts had just discussed my case that morning and it was unanimous for surgery. Fiddling around with treatments would just increase the risk of spread.

Dad asked, *"But what about the Keytruda?"*

Dr Chart said he had arranged for another specialist to speak to us shortly about that and then took his leave.

I turned and growled at Dad, *"You questioning it just makes it harder for me to accept it, I feel wrong for accepting it!"*

My decision was still raw, and if Dad couldn't accept and love me the way I was going to look, no one would! I really needed a united front against this hideous disease and it felt like we were divided, I was fighting two battles, one to be accepted and the other was for my life. Dad was still in denial and he struggled the most to accept the outcome. Not because he was ashamed, but he was just trying to protect his little girl. At the time I didn't see that.

A new doctor entered, his high energy filled the room instantly. His warm handshake and smile was infectious as he introduced himself I had already named him Dr Energiser. He was a stark contrast to Dr Chart; this man was curious, talkative and driven. He took the time to explain the doctors' meeting that morning, and emphasised the consideration undertaken by all. There were thirty people in the room all with very valuable input. He wanted me to be able to understand and trust the system behind the surgery. Every possible option had been explored. He was fast-talking yet captivating.

Dr Energiser was also the first to really concede that the operation was a big operation not just physically but cosmetically as well. He could see my hesitance for the surgery wasn't because I didn't want to survive, but rather fear of the adversity such a change would reap. Tears rolled down my cheeks in appreciation, I finally felt like I didn't have to fight to be understood.

He talked us through the risks of trying immunotherapy as it could be three months waiting for results from slow reacting immune cells, and not necessarily good results either. This in turn would allow time for further growth of the current melanoma cells.

He added that the alternative treatments were something we still might need down the track anyway. I hadn't considered the chance of other cancer appearing later. I might need a backup plan.

Dad persisted with the treatment questions until finally I was straight as an arrow, *"That's playing with my life … it's not happening, plain and simple."*

But Dad needed one final question answered. *"If you had a daughter in this situation, what would you do?"*

The reply was swift, *"I would do the surgery – to maximise long-term survival … You have an impressive daughter, you should be so proud."*

Despite this Dad still struggled to let the options go and I had to sideline my frustrations with him because no matter how he felt, my decision had crystallised and my goal was to live. And to live positively.

~ D Day ~

In the weeks leading up to the surgery I was on an emotional rollercoaster, trying to continue living my normal life working and socialising. Nights were filled with tears and fears, days spent either yelling or not talking at all. I escaped a lot with my friends and drowned my sorrows with alcohol, pretending I was making the most of my time before surgery while in reality it was to quieten the anxiety beneath the surface so I could feel like a normal carefree 22-year-old.

Outwardly I was dealing with it all so well, logically understanding why this needed to happen. But that logical mind wasn't always there and then I would rant and scream that it was unfair! I was scared to let out the raw emotion I felt because I didn't think my friends would want to stay in the picture if they saw my tears. A small part of me agonised how long would their support and love last post-surgery, would they want to be seen in public with me once I actually did look different?

I had opted for counselling after all and it even benefited my family as they all went to see the counsellor separately too. It was a tough time on so many levels. Mum and Dad were finding their way as parents of a sick young adult, sharing a desired outcome and needing to come together as a team, despite being divorced and living in different countries. I so admire the way they dealt with this difficult situation, having to support each other while keeping their own feelings of hurt to the side.

While for me, being able to unload my feelings onto an objective listener was such a relief, knowing my words wouldn't impact their life. Even before the cancer started, I had long been accustomed to being the rock in my family, the delegator, the organiser and I was scared that my inability to support and help them would see the family crumble when I couldn't maintain this role through the dark times ahead.

I planned my last week with care, lots of self-care. A make-up course, retail therapy and searching out inspiring stories and motivational speakers. I wasn't alone in adversity and I had the power to control my experience by learning from people who had lived through it already.

The hurdles started coming at me. Firstly, I had to sign the consent papers for the surgery to happen – they called it elective surgery! That was a hard pill to swallow. Then I thought visiting my recovery ward would be a good idea, I wanted to know if they could adhere to the guidelines for AYA (Adolescence and Young Adults) care. I explained to the senior nurse that I wanted one of my parents to stay with me after the surgery.

She simply burst into laughter and mocked me. *"How old do you think you are? Seriously we let that happen with children but you're an adult."*

I was so fragile. I didn't feel like an adult at all! *"I'm not really, I'm only 22, I still live at home and I just need them here supporting me while I go through the toughest surgery of my life."*

She practically spat back at me, *"At 22 you're legally an adult so don't be ridiculous, you can get through this on your own."*

I didn't know what else to say, my courage left me, I felt alone. Was I acting like a child? Was needing my parents during this time pathetic? I had always been independent, but a lot of that was because I knew they had my back.

I left feeling like cancer was stealing my identity, surrounded by anxiety again and the fear of being alone. I had relied on a sense of peace that my parents would always be near me through the trials to come. I practically ran to my counsellor's room nearby, and let it out. I cried and cried like I was grieving all over again with another unwelcome change. She gently reminded me I had the strength to handle whatever happened on the day.

At 6 am on Friday October 9, 2015. My mum, brother and two sisters clambered into the car as we drove to the hospital for my surgery, Dad would meet us there. Nobody talked; there was no backing down. My mind became still and quiet. My sister, Brittany on the other-hand was her typical crazy self. She kept telling me how cool it would be to watch the surgery, she wanted to ask the medical staff if she could be in there with me and keep my eye in a glass jar afterwards. I wasn't too impressed with her eye jokes at the time, I was laser-focused. I had tunnel vision to accomplish only one mission — to get through this life-saving surgery, I'd deal with the repercussions afterwards. I just had to get through it first.

My other siblings and my parents were a little overwhelmed, we were all a bit confronted and out of our depths, our reactions and emotions of dealing with this unique situation were as different as we were, but there was an underlying feeling of fierce loyalty which held me steady.

I was an observer as I put on my surgical gown and watched the preparation go on around me. A haze, a blur surrounded me.

We clutched together as a family and the mood heightened.

Mum spontaneously burst into laughter as I was getting ready. *What was so funny?* Mum was laughing so hard and grabbing for her camera. My navy-blue undies had the words — 'LETS PARTY!' — printed in fluoro-pink right across the bum. We laughed hysterically at the inappropriateness of the words plastered across my backside. This definitely wasn't a party.

Mum did what any over-protective and respectful mother would do and posted it to straight to Facebook! And our "fundies tradition" had begun! I figured from then on, if I had to have surgery, I might as well do it my way, in Jess-style. Fundies and all.

As the moment got nearer and the laughter subsided, I soon found myself in a daze, as we slowly made our way to the surgical prep area. The nurses asked questions, took my temperature and my blood pressure (which was very high). I was lost in my own head, and while I could see people around me moving and fussing, it was like the world was on mute. All I could hear was my own thoughts.

I had done my best to mentally, emotionally and physically prepare, I had a collection of eyepatches in my bag ready for their debut, but there was no guarantee I was going to hold up on the other side. I tried to imagine it, I tried to visualise my strength and courage, standing proud on the other side, but all I could see was me sitting in a room alone, with one eye. I didn't look sad or down, but I also didn't look confident. I looked numb, and maybe that's what I'd become. I tried to push those images aside as I was wheeled into surgery.

With long hugs and sounds of good luck, my parents wheeled my bed toward the surgical doors. I kissed goodbye the last familiar faces I would see with both eyes.

The next faces would be my medical team and the man I trusted with my life. I prayed I was leaving behind my life with cancer and that going through these surgical doors meant a new life; one of unknown challenges but more importantly possibility.

Hope can be a lifesaver and I clutched it with all my might.

~ The Waiting Game ~

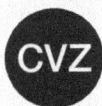

Craig Van Zeil
9 October 2015

Jess went in for surgery this morning and her operation was a success and went according to plan. The Dr confirmed the lump under her eye was indeed a Melanoma, so the operation was the correct procedure. She is in a lot of pain, but is getting a lot of attention from the nurses who will bring it under control. She will be in hospital for about 3 days. I do not see this as an operation to remove her eye, but rather as a procedure to save her from a vicious and aggressive form of cancer. I cannot tell you how proud I am of my Jess, having the strength of her conviction to make this very hard, life-changing decision. She had to make this decision on her own as this decision will last her for the rest of her life. Jess has been so resolute and positive about this decision and has never wavered that this was the right thing to do. As her Dad I kept looking at options in a desperate effort to prevent this procedure from happening. But Jess somehow knew this was the right decision and after all my searching and researching, I had to agree with her and am even more convinced now that the operation is done. This is the only option to give her the best chance of a cancer-free life going forward.

Jess and I have chatted a lot and at length over time leading up to this procedure and all I kept reminding Jess is that no matter what happens on the outside, no one can take away her special heart, her spirit and her soul.

I believe that in life things happen for a reason. I believe that Jess will look back at some time in the future and realise that she has achieved new heights and will be doing things that would never have been possible if she had not gone through this. I don't know a stronger person who will turn this into something so positive in her life.

I want to thank everyone who has donated and still wants to donate to the cause that Britt put together for Jess called Eye-won. This money will be used to help Jess rehabilitate and get her life back to normality. I appreciate the kindness that so many people have shown to Jess. Thank you.

If you still want to contribute towards Jess's rehabilitation, just click on the link and you can make a donation on your VISA card from any country. *https://www.mycause.com.au/page/110647/eye-won*

I now ask that you all rally around Jess and help her get back into normal life. If you see her around, don't be nervous to approach her as she needs all your support and is in a good frame of mind about this decision.

Thanks again for the endless support from everyone, it really is appreciated.

Please feel free to post and re post this so everyone is kept up to speed with Jess.

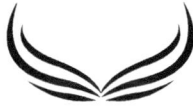

CHAPTER 6

A NEW WORLD

"Because one believes in oneself, one doesn't try to convince others. Because one is content with oneself, one doesn't need others' approval. Because one accepts oneself, the whole world accepts him or her."

— *Lao Tzu*

I woke up slowly and painfully in recovery, I could sense my mum nearby. I was burning up and in agony. I vomited profusely which only increased the pain. I slipped in and out of consciousness; asking for my dad and when I blinked again there he was. I panicked because none of this pain was easing. For two days I was either sleeping, eating, vomiting or zonked out on medications and talking gibberish.

There were so many tiny challenges to get through each initial moment. I needed a ridiculous amount of pain medication and barely slept at all. As I gained my equilibrium, I knew I was so blessed to have so many friends and family members come and visit me in hospital bearing lots of delicious treats.

Then came the morning when they would remove my bandages. I would look in the mirror for the first time, post-surgery. I was terrified, and burning with anticipation. The nurse and the doctor were both young females. They made this intimate process beautiful and one I will remember forever. They were gentle and nurturing and made me feel so comfortable when moments earlier I had wanted to lock myself in the bathroom and leave the bandage on for good.

There was no noise as it fell away, no loud false exclamations. Just gentle encouraging smiles. I almost bounded out of bed to see my new face. I expected to see someone foreign staring back at me, but I saw my bright familiar smile, my freckled cheeks, my button nose, my on-point eyebrows. The only difference: there was one eye staring back not two.

I analysed my face and saw a soft beauty in it, my smile brightened as I accepted the woman in the mirror as me. I silently told her she was beautiful, that she was strong, courageous and still me. I tried out some eyepatches and explored the world a little, embracing my new fashion accessory. The doctors were pleased with my recovery and when I left the hospital a few days later my friend Liv sprinkled glitter over me as I crossed the threshold, a christening to my new

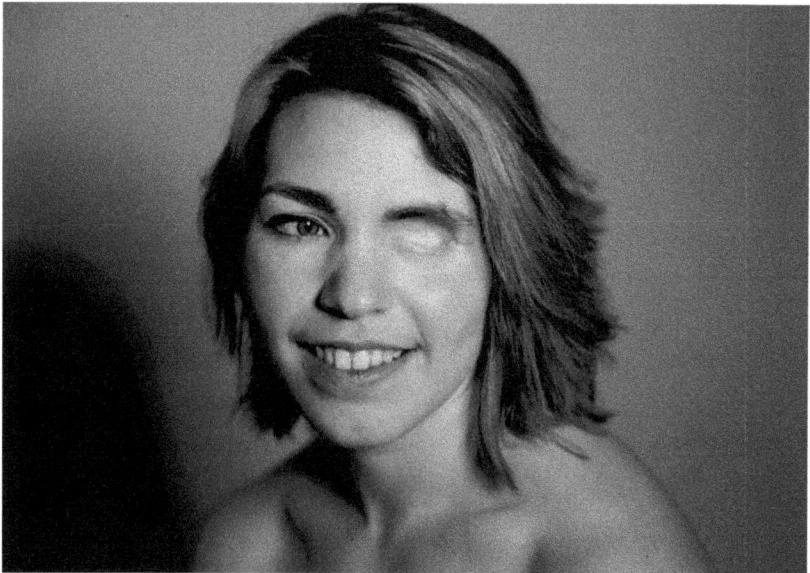

Taken 10 months after surgery.

sparkly life.

After a few days of settling in at home my body was still adjusting to monocular living. It was tiring, but I pushed my brain to get used to the new depth perception by pouring glasses of water and bouncing a tennis ball against a wall and catching it. The more I practised the faster new neural pathways would be created and therefore the faster I could start back at the things I loved.

Only ten days after surgery I was driving for the first time. Dad gave me no choice but to get behind the wheel. He knew that if I didn't do it soon, it would only become harder to break through the fear. I was terrified getting behind the wheel, what if something went wrong, what if I'd forgotten how to drive? But as I drove down the familiar roads it felt natural, nothing had really changed.

Getting back to work a little over a month later was both exciting and challenging. My independence returned but physically I was still exhausted. I needed to nap for twice as long as my shift was.

The first of the confronting experiences also began. During one of my shifts at the Kid's Activity Centre I worked at, I was drawn to help a mother whose young daughter was crying. Before I could enquire whether I could help, the lady cut over the top of me exclaiming loudly, *"Look at the pirate, isn't she scary!"*

I felt like an animal in a zoo! She was happy to disregard my feelings in an attempt to distract her child. It became starkly obvious to me that such a naive, insensitive attitude to adversity can impact a child's outlook on life. It teaches children that it's OK to point out people's flaws and so begin the cycle of mistreating one another or even bullying.

In reality, the first year was hard, every day I put on a patch and a big bright smile, but it used to hit hard when people down the street would stare, point or loudly make fun of me for being a pirate or weird.

Being different, and standing out was an adjustment, there were days where I felt proud and there were days I wanted to avoid people all together. On my good days I could brush it off but when I was already feeling self-conscious or ashamed it just ripped me down. Tears would well up, I'd find myself staring at the ground and trying to hide.

Eventually, I realised it actually didn't matter what they thought. I didn't want to be associated with people who would judge me before they had even spoken to me. I was proud of the person I had become, the things I had overcome and the way I looked! Yes, it was different, I did stand out but this was me now. I stopped noticing other people's actions and started focusing on me and how I could become the person I knew I wanted to be.

We should praise people who have risen above their adversity, looking up to their bravery and strength. Society should not be so quick to judge and label disabilities. I dream of creating an open and accepting generation where no one is cast aside for their abnormalities, everyone is different and differences should be celebrated!

~ Running Uphill ~

I was excited to return to my studies in the New Year, back to things that brought me joy and challenged me. Studying was a lot harder than I had expected, I loved the units but they required a lot of study time. Long hours at the computer put incredible strain on my eye, add in the long travel time and I fell into bed at night by 6.30pm, often with a chronic migraine. Gradually my stamina increased and I kept at it. My results were really great that semester and I was loving what I was learning more than ever.

Three months after the surgery Dr Chart was pleased to see the scans showed everything was looking great and recovering well internally. Dr Watch was pleased with how the scar and the socket were recovering externally, and even more pleased to see me laughing, smiling and rocking such a colourful eyepatch.

In May 2016 I had my second scans since the surgery, Dr Chart was astounded to see that there were no signs of melanoma anywhere. He decided to push my scans out to being every 6 months right then. This decision didn't sit well with me, I was meant to be scanning regularly for the first 12 months, but he was the expert and I did trust him.

Six months after the surgery I was back at the gym and running almost every day, I fell in love with the freedom of running on my local trails and along the beachfront. I had set myself a goal of running my first half marathon by the end of 2016. I also booked a trip to New Zealand and planned to hike the Milford Sound in March 2017. My life was filled with adventurous plans; dreams that made my heart sing.

As healthy as I was feeling, in June I started getting abdominal pain and bloating, I started reacting to all sorts of food and could hardly eat. I lost ten kilos and was diagnosed with severe IBS. I was put on a low FODMAP diet which counts out a lot of different foods and it all began to make sense. I was uneasy about the weight loss and struggled to put it back on again. As soon as I regained enough strength I returned to running. Sometimes my right leg would turn to jelly mid-run, and I'd have to stop and shake it out for five minutes. This was a signal that I couldn't have recognised. I blamed it on the increased exercise and challenges of getting enough calories from the diet I had to maintain.

By September 2016, eleven months after losing my eye I had fully embraced my journey. In honour of the one year 'Eye-aversary' coming up, I wanted to celebrate the loss that had in turn saved my entire life, by throwing an eye-themed party!

This particular morning both Mum and myself were home sitting around the table together. Me, on the pretence of studying while Mum was legitimately working from home, a rare occurrence indeed. In actual fact, a good friend's brother had sadly passed away while overseas and Mum had planned to accompany me to the funeral. However, there was a delay in returning the body to Australia, and the funeral had to be postponed at the last minute, leaving Mum home unexpectedly.

My discarded assignment was replaced with endless chatter about banners and balloons. Eventually I could see Mum had had her fill of eye-themed decorations and wanted to get back to her work so I sauntered off to shower.

Later as I dried my feet I noticed the small toe on my right foot twitching and bouncing. I watched a few moments waiting for it to stop but it only began to twitch more vigorously.

"Mum? Can you come here?" I called out.

Mum grumbled away from her work towards the bathroom as my toes kept up their tremors. She wasn't alarmed when she saw it, *"Jess, it's just a twitch, relax."*

But as the words left her mouth the twitch changed and my whole foot started to pulsate, my toes stretched out and then curled back in perfect synchronicity. My stomach dropped and I felt light-headed.

My whole calf muscle had joined the party by now, Mum thought it was a cramp and that I was winding myself up but I knew it wasn't. It looked as though there was an invisible hand grabbing and squeezing my calf as if it was putty. I yelled back that it wasn't a cramp! She helped me sit down onto the floor when suddenly I felt a surge of electricity through my entire right leg and up into my body.

"Jess! Do you need me to call an ambulance?!"

I could hear and see Mum clearly but I couldn't breathe to respond, someone was sitting on my chest, I was choking on my own words! I panicked, 'What if she doesn't call the ambulance, what if she doesn't know anything is wrong?!' As my vision started to blur the last thing I remember was thinking, 'How ironic, I survived cancer and now I'm going to die of a heart attack!'

I woke up terrified and confused; had I been out of it for days? I scrambled to sit up in pure panic. *"Jess, it's OK, stay still, the paramedics will be here soon."* I had so many questions but all I could do was sob into Mum's arms. *"I thought I was dying, I never expected to wake up!"*

She held me tight and whispered, *"So did I."*

The paramedics were amazing. I felt bombarded with questions and checks but I knew that was necessary. They thought it sounded like a seizure and as it was my first one, it was protocol to admit me to hospital. They saw my panicked face and assured me they'd just do some scans to ensure it was all fine. Those words sound scary out of context but at the time, they calmed me down, validating what I had gone through was worth investigating. More than that, it meant it hadn't been a heart attack or a stroke, that maybe it was epilepsy and while that wasn't ideal it also wasn't life threatening.

Mum and I were back to the old waiting game once we got to the hospital. Mum shared her experience of those intense moments during the seizure and it must have been excruciating for her. My arms had flailed about wildly and then I went still and grey; she thought I was dead. The emergency operator calmed her down to check my chest closely for signs of breathing and she could see it moving minutely. She put me in the recovery position and kept me warm. I cannot imagine what it was like to think her daughter was dying in front of her eyes and feel so helpless. I realised if she hadn't been home that day, I might have fallen and hit my head. It could have been so much worse and I still thank my guardian angel up there who arranged for my mum to be home with me that day.

Over the course of a few hours I was sent for a brain CT and then an MRI. We'd been at the hospital for so long with no food or real contact with my siblings that Mum ducked home for supplies while waiting for the results. The female doctor I'd met before my scans found me while Mum was gone; her eyes darted around the room and she looked a little distressed. She was disappointed when I explained that Mum wasn't there.

"It's OK, you can talk to me without a parent."

Instead she replied, "I know but I think it best we wait."

She asked me to let the nurse know when Mum returned and she left me there with no support for my increasing level of panic. I called Mum's mobile repeatedly, by the time she answered I was hysterical, yelling at her for not answering her phone, for leaving me, because no one would tell me what was going on until she was back. It was the fear talking and I know it was hard for her to listen to me like that; both annoyed at me and worried herself.

My Mum returned looking flustered and irritated with the way I'd spoken to her. This situation was setting us both on edge, the unknown, the fears, the waiting, the stress; it was all a bit much for a Friday afternoon. When the doctor returned to see us, I could see her face was strained.

"The reason I want you both here is because we found out what caused the seizure." There was a long anxious pause. "It's the melanoma, it has metastasised to your brain."

The doctor's head hung low in sympathy as though she was handing me my death sentence. Mum buckled over and started wailing, the news seemed to break her. My heart sunk to see their reactions.

Yet somehow, I felt calm and at peace, a gentle but authoritative voice filled my head. "It's not your time. Yes, it's going to be a tough journey ahead BUT you still have so much to offer this world. This will not be the end."

From thinking my boxing match was over, I was being hauled back in the ring for a climactic round two. My prognosis was estimated at this point between 6-16 weeks but I didn't register this possibility; I was not going to be a statistic.

I took a huge breath; I believed those inner words I'd heard to my core. Now was not the time for emotions, I needed to get my game plan in place.

"OK. That's not ideal. What's next, how do we move forward from here?"

The doctor was surprised at my composure but explained I'd be monitored here for 24 hours then transferred to my treating hospital, Peter Mac; which meant Dr Energiser.

"OK. Good. That sounds like a good plan. Thank you."

Mum and I sat in silence for a moment before we leapt into action, calling family, friends and anyone else who needed to know first-hand. It wasn't easy but I was in a very technical mode called, 'GET SHIT DONE' mode and that meant putting my emotions to the side for now. It hurt like hell each time I told someone and heard their distraught tears but I had to keep it together.

My Dad was amazing. He was back in the country within 24 hours. My gorgeous girlfriends came in at separate times claiming to be my sisters, the nurses were understanding and turned a blind eye.

This was the toughest 24 hours of my journey so far, yet rising above that was the knowledge I had never felt more loved or supported than I did that day. I was living in a state of gratitude. I focused on all the hidden blessings; that Mum had been unusually home to help me, the efficiency of the '000' Operator, the comfort from the paramedics, the fabulous nurses, the doctor waiting for my mum to break the news, my dad flying over so fast, the list goes on.

~ The Cost of a Life ~

Once I'd been transferred to the new hospital, my room in the ward was big, beautiful and private, with a sofa bed to allow someone to stay with me at all times. Faced with all the uncertainty around me, this environment helped me stay calm; panicking wouldn't help me, the best thing was to look after myself for the time being. I knew the team here would do everything they could for me. After a quiet weekend, Monday bustled with activity and it was a relief to see Dr Energiser again with his familiar smile and enthusiasm.

He gave me the information straight up. They had found several tumours on my brain. The one on the motor cortex (in charge of movement) had haemorrhaged and was the cause of the seizure. First up was brain surgery to remove the 'problem spot', which would hopefully stop any more seizures. This would need to happen within the week.

Next was the problem of the six or so other tiny tumours that were visible on the scan but were inoperable due to their locations. Three were in the frontal lobe (which controls personality, language, behaviour, expression) and three or four were near the cerebellum (helps with coordination, balance and speech).

This meant I would need another form of treatment to hopefully shrink and kill the visible tumours but also eradicate any other cancerous cells that may have seeded but were not yet visible on the scans. Dr Energiser explained that they were having big discussions about my case again to work out what that treatment option would look like; they were considering immunotherapy (the drugs my dad was so excited by the first time around) which now had more options available than just Keytruda, as well as considering radiation, either whole brain or targeted radiation.

I had been listening openly until that point, keen to get a plan in place. When I heard *radiation*, I went white as a sheet. I was desperate to avoid radiation. I was passionate about my career path as a speaker and I didn't want to risk radiation affecting the wrong part of my brain. Not to mention how much I had learnt to love the person I had become that radiation could alter. These were my own fears and perceptions of what I thought radiation could do rather than medical advice.

Dr Energiser understood but stressed the situation may need it. I did trust him but reiterated if there was any way to avoid it, I wanted to.

Two more teams of doctors came to see me. I learnt about the risks of surgery and that it could result in me losing the ability to walk. I felt a shiver of fear run through me. The risks could seem overwhelming if you let them. They couldn't give me a date or time, just that the surgery would be soon; it terrified me.

When the radiation oncology team arrived, I closed off mentally. They answered my questions eloquently and said how much it could help. But they were my last option and I made that clear.

That evening I was exhausted. My life in the space of a few days had been thrown into a whirlwind of medical jargon and major decisions that could impact my life forever or even risk me not being here.

That night Dad and I were woken by a team of people at 10.30pm. I was being moved to the hospital across the road so that I was already admitted when it was time for the surgery. What? I was so groggy and confused; this was so much sooner than I could deal with! Not to mention the ridiculous notion of waking us and moving us in the middle of the night! Dad railed loudly that we needed time to come to terms with the surgery, but time was something we didn't have. Once again, I felt out of control in my own life. One of the orderlies said simply, *"You need this surgery, if you don't come with us now they will drop your priority listing."*

What else could we do? We scurried around collecting my things and moved into the nearby hospital where the surgery would happen. It was older, darker and much gloomier. We tried to settle in quietly but we were in an open ward with other patients and kept getting hushed by the staff. A nurse tried to tell Dad he couldn't stay but he stood his ground because there was no way he could get home at 12.30! I was miserable and scared and couldn't contemplate not seeing my mum before the surgery; I needed to be held by her one last time. Dad and I didn't sleep that night with all the disturbances; he comforted my worries and little cries of distress. I hated this new hospital, I hated the sounds, the lack of privacy but more than anything I hated how it made me feel like a prisoner to my own disease, a number not a person.

Morning meant more noise and disturbances and this place looked even drearier in the light. Mum arrived a little after 9am, to find me in a 'hangry', short tempered and irritable state. They didn't have my dietary needs listed and I couldn't eat what the meal staff had brought around. Finally catching the nurse's attention to explain, she wasn't bothered at all because apparently, I was listed as fasting before surgery anyway – just great – anything else I was not going to be told?!

Hours passed and there were no answers to when this surgery might be, or most importantly when the hell I could eat. In this place, I just felt like a number in the system that was frequently forgotten about, everyone seemed to know what was going on for me but they didn't feel the need to extend these plans to me. I was also confined to the stuffy ward as I was on the waiting list for surgery; this place was getting worse and worse.

When Dr Energiser arrived, I blurted out my frustration over the debacle of the previous evening, not being told the surgery was imminent and how I hated it here! While compassionate enough to explain there would have been a good reason for the disruptions, he didn't have any answers and had come to talk about our next steps after the surgery.

Another multi-specialist meeting that morning had discussed my case; with neurosurgeons, medical oncologists, surgical oncologists and radiation oncologists. They had narrowed treatment down to two immunotherapy options.

First was Keytruda which was fully funded by the PBS (Pharmaceutical Benefit Scheme) and usually has a 25-30% response rate. However, they noted my rare mutation type of melanoma doesn't seem to respond as readily.

The other was a dual treatment, meaning two treatments used in tandem called Ipilimumab and Nivolumab. Nivolumab works in a similar manner to Keytruda and the Ipilimumab compliments it, increasing response rates to approximately 55%. This is the only treatment they'd had great success with for my specific mutation.

Dr Energiser paused, his usual passion seemed drained. There were two issues to face with this treatment he explained; the first was that with the increased response rate we would also see an increase in side effects, 75% of all patients suffered side effects on this treatment.

The second was that this drug was not yet on the PBS, meaning it will have to be self-funded. The treatment would cost around $30,000 per dose and I would need four doses, unless the side effects got too severe in which case I would have to stop treatment early and be put onto steroids.

My jaw dropped, the treatment was going to cost $120,000!

"Well we're going to have to go with the Keytruda, there is no way we can afford the dual treatment." I stammered.

In unison my parents responded forcefully, *"Jess, this is your life we're talking about – we'll find the money!"*

Tears were streaming down my face, *"I'm not letting you spend that kind of money on me, to put yourselves in financial jeopardy for a treatment that may or may not work when there is one that's free that could also work."*

It was no time for delicacy, I continued angrily. *"What if it doesn't work and I die and all you have left is a huge debt and no daughter to show for it – then what? I can't let you. It's not happening. This is my life, my treatment, my choice and I'm saying no!"*

My parents stared back with tear-filled eyes as if I had betrayed them.

Dr Energiser looked at me steadily, *"If there is any way you can afford the treatment I would highly suggest it, it has the greatest chance of getting you through this."*

I was infuriated; not only did I have to fight the tumours but I now felt the insult of being charged for the privilege. *"It's a 50/50 chance, literally a toss of a coin. Spending that kind of money is literally gambling and it's not like we get double or nothing – my parents either get their daughter or I die."* I spat back bitterly.

Dr Energiser knew the bitterness wasn't directed at him and responded with a stern tone, *"You have tumours on the brain Jess and that's not a place you want melanoma, it's very hard to treat and we have limited options. But you are lucky we actually have some options open to us. You have options that could save your life and you need to make the best decision that you and your family can live with and you need to make it soon."*

With that he walked out, leaving a broken family behind him.

As my parents bickered over my bed, I had never felt closer to death than I did in that moment. I was distraught to think I had to make a decision on my life that could financially break my family. My life had a dollar value and I didn't know if I was willing to take the gamble on it and see if it paid off.

The incredible side story to all this, is the battle my divorced parents overcame to support me as a unit through this time. Spending almost every waking hour supporting their daughter, their other children, processing my diagnosis, finding 100k for my treatment, keeping their individual businesses running while operating on stress and sleep deprivation. Not surprisingly there was tension, hushed arguments and some little outbursts. I can only imagine how hard it all was as a divorced couple and I have immense gratitude to them for rising above it all so we could unite to make it through this war zone together.

It was a heartwrenching conversation for all of us. I still felt the financial burden was too much.

"But Jess it's my money, our money, and if you don't let us try and then you die we will always wonder." Mum fought on through tears. *"And if we do try and it doesn't work then at least we will know we gave it our best shot, we gave you every chance there was. We'll know that we never ever gave up on you."*

I slumped over feeling helpless.

Finally, Dad looked up and said, *"Well what if we fundraise? Would you take the treatment then?"*

I caught his eye and for the first time that day I felt hope, my lips trembled in a small smile. *"That's a lot of money to fundraise Dad."* I could see his mind racing.

"Leave it to me."

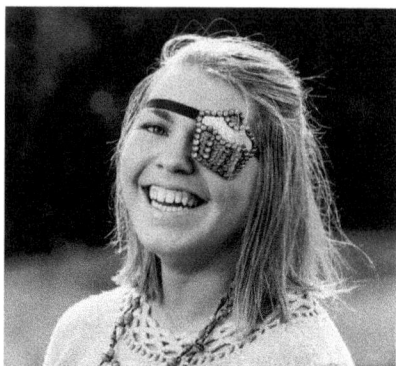
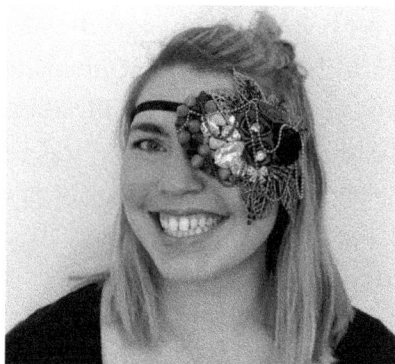
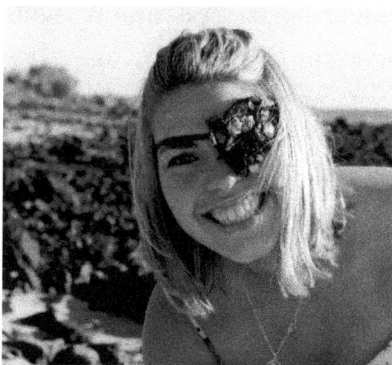
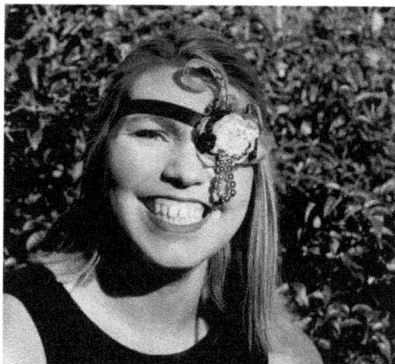
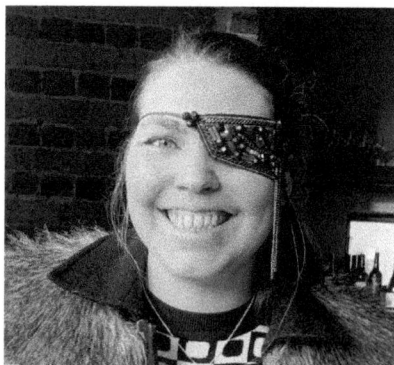
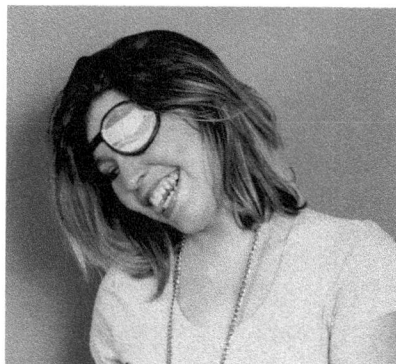

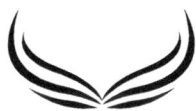

CHAPTER 7

BRAIN SURGERY

*"I can be changed by what happens to me. But I
refuse to be reduced by it."*
— *Maya Angelou*

My mood lifted with that dose of hope. We had a plan in place and fundraising could be a real option. The unexpected kept occurring though and at 4pm, the nurse told me I could break my fast because I would not be in for surgery until Friday now. I was beyond infuriated that I could have been happily staying in my lovely old room this whole time, it all felt like a joke at my expense! Mum was quickly rummaging through my snack bag because she sensed half this pent-up anger was because I was ravenous! This nurse was very empathetic, apologising for the stress and explaining that it happened sometimes.

We do have a fantastic medical system here in Australia, but sometimes there are cracks that seem deeply engrained. When you feel like a number being tossed around needlessly, this insensitivity produces an inordinate amount of stress that seems avoidable. I always went above and beyond to treat the wonderful staff with love, patience and respect, but some of my biggest challenges in hospital came from the system failing and my patience was tested.

The following morning the news came that I was being discharged. What?! Apparently I was 'under control', I hadn't had a seizure since I'd started on medication and there was no reason for me to be kept in when I didn't have to be. I just needed to be here by 6am Friday morning for surgery.

This created a dilemma, I was happy to think of a full night's sleep but utterly terrified I might have another seizure with no one around. I blurted my fears out to the nurse and listed other reasons to stay in my safety bubble that I had so recently claimed to hate.

The nurse conceded I could stay if I wanted to but also that it would be a good time to really rest before surgery, assuring me I wouldn't have been discharged unless they were sure it was safe. When a good friend of Mum's offered us to stay in her city apartment, we accepted.

Before we left, Dr Energiser came to talk again about treatments and was really pleased we had decided to go forward with the dual treatment. *"We just need 12,000 people to donate $10, that's so doable!"* His smile spread ear to ear at my excitement.

This didn't last though. *"So what do the statistics say about Jess's chance of survival?"* Dad was in rational mode and I really did not appreciate it. Dr Energiser did his best and answered honestly, he said there just wasn't the data or studies to provide any statistics on this rare situation we were in. He just knew this treatment would give me the best chance to keep fighting.

Dad was like a terrier and wouldn't give up.

"But how long will it give her? Does it guarantee her at least a year, 2 years, 5 years, her whole life?" I was glaring angrily at Dad but he wasn't paying attention. Again, the doctor conceded that besides good short-term results, he didn't know.

"But if you were to give it a guess, how long would you say it would give her?"

Steam was coming out of my ears by now.

Dr Energiser was driven to explaining that he couldn't just make up an answer.

Dad went to intercede again but I cut him off. *"Dad! He cannot give us a response because there isn't data to base it on, which is a good thing because I don't want to know."*

Dad looked at me puzzled, *"But an indication of something would be good ..."*

"Only if it's a good statistic but not if my chance of survival is 2% – I don't want to know that!"

"But these are the questions we should be asking."

"DAD! Regardless of whether Dr Energiser can give you statistics – I don't want to know! I am not going to base my hope, my efforts and my recovery on a statistic. I don't want to be focused on them, I am not just another number on a data sheet; my life is more than that. So, stop!"

Dr Energiser wasn't fazed by the familial disagreement. He smiled as he left, wishing me luck until he saw me again in recovery.

We still had to unravel our disagreement and it was challenging to understand and respect our views. Dad wasn't impressed with the public put down but I was adamant the way I wanted to handle it. It was my treatment, my illness and if I didn't want to know the statistics then I shouldn't have to. He was more than welcome to ask in private but as there were things I did not want to know he should respect that.

He looked hurt and explained this information would help manage our expectations.

Mum sighed and argued for me, *"Craig, Jess is right, if she doesn't want to know the statistics of whether she will survive, she shouldn't have to. Frankly I agree with her and don't want to know either, she is not saying don't ask but you can ask in private."*

Dad looked at us in disbelief, *"This is ridiculous, I'm just trying to do what I think is right!"*

He had absolutely been supporting me as much as humanly possible but no one's perfect and Dad struggled to contain his need to control and question everything. He'd had enough and stormed out leaving Mum and I in shock.

It was a surreal stage to play out much of our family's saga, emotions, grudges and misunderstandings from the past. I was 16 when Dad left, a time when I still needed guidance and parenting.

I had grown so much since then but elements of our relationship hadn't evolved to reflect this and he probably expected to have as much influence as he did have before. Now all he wanted was to arm us all with every known statistic to protect his daughter. We all got pretty edgy at times, but either way I had my calm, nurturing Mum, and my proactive Dad looking out for me in the storm.

~ Rest and Worry ~

Mum and I made a mad dash for the car in fear that someone would change their minds and tell us we needed to stay. The apartment was the perfect retreat from the hospital noises and I fell instantly asleep. Those two days were as relaxing as they could be, walking in the fresh air, shopping, eating out and seeing friends and family.

It was a beautiful time, where I relaxed and enjoyed some normal living, but the nights were the hardest. Although I was exhausted I had so much playing on my mind, I refused to sleep on my own in case I had a seizure so Mum shared a bed with me. The quiet of the nights let my deep thoughts, my fears and loneliness in.

I might never walk again, but then again, I was so incredibly lucky to be here. Although the seizure was by far one of the my most challenging and emotional experiences, it was also a blessing because it meant we had detected the melanoma early enough that it hadn't spread to the rest of my body, that it was still treatable, that I still had a chance at life after cancer!

On Friday morning the dreaded alarm went off at 4.45am. My heart seemed to beat out of my chest, I was trying to look calm for my mum's sake but I was irritable and terrified.

Neither of us really spoke on the way there. I was going through all the potential outcomes, reminding myself that even if I ended up in a wheelchair I could lead a full and amazing life. I thought of a boy I knew from primary school who had ended up in a wheelchair; he'd just completed a study semester abroad and his life was amazing. I was determined to do the same if that was my fate.

Once again, I found myself filling in an, 'elective surgery' form. I scoffed and mumbled, *"I hardly think I am electing to have brain surgery, I need it or I'll die."*

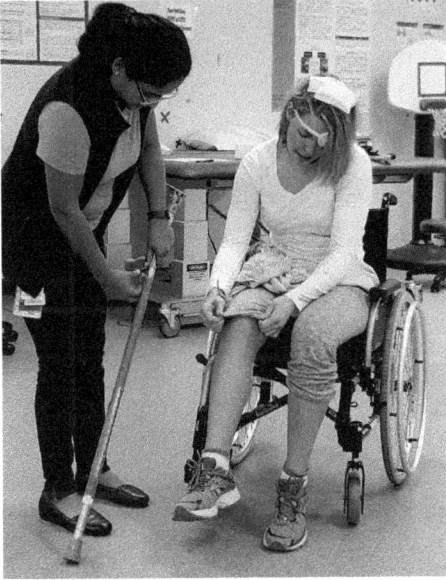

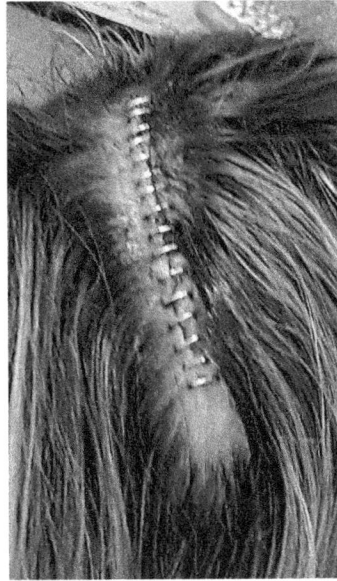

I was grateful the lady took the time to answer kindly, *"I know you wouldn't choose this darling, it's just a legal form that says you are capable of accepting the surgery, that we haven't had to take action with no response."* They really should change the name of that form.

My cheer squad arrived and I could feel their apprehension but also the love and care. I had thrown on my fundies again to bring some humour to such an intense moment. I opted for Wonder Woman, after all she is seriously awesome and known for fighting evil. Although I didn't have an invisible jet or the Lasso of Truth, I could carry her fearless attitude and fight my own battle. I had to.

Thankfully, my argument with Dad was forgotten as everyone huddled around me. Britt teased me, wondering why I wouldn't be awake for the surgery as that would be way cooler in her opinion!

When I heard my name, it was time for a teary goodbye to my siblings. My parents could come along to the examination rooms where I was seen by numerous doctors as they ticked their official boxes. The last two doctors got the brunt of my irritation, after being poked, prodded, questioned and examined for almost two hours — I was over it.

When I was asked for the sixth time, did I understand the risks that there's a 5% chance I'll never regain movement on the right side and a much higher chance I'll have reduced function on that side, I lost it.

"I get it! I get there's a risk with the surgery and I've accepted them but when all of you keep reminding me it doesn't make it any easier, it makes me terrified of the surgery and I don't have a choice, I have to have it, it's this surgery or my life!"

The young doctor just stuttered, *"Well legally we have to tell you."*

"If you want me in that surgery then this is the last time!" The young doctors hurried it up after that.

Another doctor prepped me for surgery and I said a final goodbye to my parents. It was surreal walking around, knowing that this could be the last time I would ever have the sensation of putting one foot in front of the other, I was reluctant to lie down because I wanted to savour a few more moments on my feet.

My surgeon, was calm, kind and extremely thorough. I was worried that I'd been told I could only have Panadol after the surgery.

"I'll make sure you aren't in pain, trust me." He gave me a wink and I instantly trusted him with my whole heart and finally felt ready for the surgery. Dr Marvel this one will be. I was keeping with my superhero theme. I figured Dr Marvel in his Spiderman scrubs and Jess in Wonder Woman underwear could take on the world.

My anaesthetist put to rest my other worry of having a reaction like last surgery; the vomiting, the pain, the fevers and the fact that I had woken up during surgeries with local anaesthetic before. He would make allowances for all previous reactions and assured me I'd wake up feeling much better than last time.

Finally, I blushed as I quickly whispered that I was in the middle of my period but the staff said it was nothing to worry about and they wouldn't be going anywhere near there, I felt like we had covered all the bases and was a little more at ease. When Dr Marvel announced they were ready for me I swallowed my last pang of fear. I counted backwards from ten and I watched the world become fuzzy before it disappeared.

~ Baby Steps ~

Post-surgery I woke feeling fit as a fiddle. I was comfortable and alert. I chatted away to the nurses taking regular obs, there were lots of physical tests. The first time a nurse asked me to squeeze her hand with my right hand, it was weak but there was a slight response, I could push and pull back gently. My face widened in hope, I was moving, I could do it!

My right foot however, did not move. I could feel her tickling me, and it was the weirdest feeling willing it to move yet it didn't even twitch, it just lay there, limp. The nurse could see the disappointment and frustration in my face as I tried over and over again to get some sort of response, she reminded me what early days it was and not to lose hope. I attempted a smile but couldn't help the thinking how easy that was to say and what would she know.

Dr Marvel announced the surgery had been a success and that he believed they got the whole tumour out! He was surprised I was so awake and responsive. He lit up with excitement too when he saw my right arm moving and responding. I was despondent about my leg but he wasn't deterred at all.

"Jess this is such a good sign! You have movement in your right side! Which means you should be able to get some if not full movement back!"

His words had given me new hope and purpose, I was going to get movement back and I knew that the sooner I could get that leg moving the better. So, from then on that's what I spent every waking hour and every ounce of energy doing. Aiming for even an inch off the bed, if I could do that I knew that everything else would be possible; walking, running and jumping would be in my grasp.

I had to spend 24 hours in the Neurosurgery intensive recovery ward getting checked regularly. Soon my parents arrived for a welcome reunion. I was still alert and chatty but every now and then I would stop mid-sentence as I focused all my energy on lifting my leg to no prevail. They were worried it was a side effect to my surgery; my tongue poking out straining in concentration. I knew my recovery depended on me getting to work straight away.

My sisters came in looking a little apprehensive, but quickly we were laughing, crying and storytelling! That damn leg still wouldn't move though.

Exhaustion set in and I dozed off. Only to be shocked awake by the alarm sounding that meant my heart rate had dropped and the nurses came at me from every angle. This happened several times like a form of sleep torture until one of the nurses realised the machine's alert was set too high with much older patients in mind.

Between the attempts to sleep and move my leg I had forgotten to ask how I'd get to the toilet if I can't move my leg? I was extremely surprised to learn they'd put in a catheter. What?! I'd been told there was nothing they needed to do below the waist! I felt my cheeks get hot and flustered, hoping they'd remembered I had my period.

I pulled up the sheets and to my horror the bed below me was covered in blood. I was so embarrassed I started to cry. I felt like I had lost all my dignity and I couldn't do anything about it. I waved Mum over and whispered it all in her ear. She asked Dad to leave the room and called the nurses over.

I was beetroot-red, asking the nurses to help me. I know it seems small, and maybe in comparison to the brain surgery, but to me in that moment I felt like a dirty caged animal rolling around in my own filth. I had had nightmares as a teenager of having my period seep through my school skirt; this was that nightmare but worse! I was embarrassed, I felt forgotten and I couldn't believe that there hadn't been any consideration in the surgery.

The nurses where so kind and understanding though; they drew the curtains and swiftly changed my sheets without having to move me, and arranged everything cleanly. They apologised that it had gone unnoticed and made me feel comfortable, like there was nothing to worry about. It was such an incredible moment for me, I felt vulnerable, embarrassed and honestly disgusted yet these two young nurses made me feel comfortable and understood.

It was that moment when I truly realised how incredible nurses are. They turned one of my most embarrassing moments into one of humility and grace, I don't know how they did it but that's the work of an earth angel.

Eight hours after surgery, somewhere amongst the cycle of dozing, check-ups and trying to move my foot, my mum was getting worried.

"Jess save your energy to recover and stop trying to move that bally leg of yours!"

I ignored her and a few tries later I let out a squeal of delight and tears of joy filled my eye! I'd done it! My leg moved off the bed just the tiniest bit but it moved! I saw so clearly a vision of me running again, crossing the finish line with a sprint. Everything felt closer; I was going to be just fine!

My smile was plastered on my face from that moment and I would show everyone around what I could do. I was proud of my persistence and of my amazing body, how blessed I am to have a body that works.

Dad came in to relieve Mum and it was a strange night indeed as we had to wake so regularly for checks. This open ward was an exceedingly strange place at 2am and we found ourselves in hysterics listening to some of the midnight mumbles of older patients. One old man a few beds down declared suddenly that he couldn't feel his head. Then he specified further, *"My head, I think I swallowed my head."* No panic – just a fact. This was one of many hilariously absurd things we heard that night. We thought to ourselves that we had the choice to laugh or cry in our situation so we may as well find the humour in it.

I was so grateful for the wonderful staff in those early hours but I can't deny that I was relieved that I'd soon be back in a normal ward. I was excited when Dr Marvel came in the next day and I could show him my new trick of moving my leg, it took a lot of energy to do but seeing his eyes light up and his smile beaming back at me with pride was amazing.

"I have no doubt you'll be up walking in no time!"

My brother Daniel, and Granny came up to give my parents a rest. I was soon moved into my new bed and I spent four days in hospital with my beautiful friends and family coming and going at all hours of the day.

It was a busy time with numerous doctors visiting, physio appointments and everything under the sun. One of the best days was when Michael Crossland, a motivational speaker I had reached out to over Instagram came and visited me while I was in hospital. We talked for a long time and at the end he helped me stand up for a photo together. This was such a humbling day and taught me an important lesson, if you want something – ask; when you have the courage to put it out there, more times than not it will happen.

~ The Lonely Path ~

Whenever I could, I would escape the ward and visit the Youth Cancer Centre across the road, or one of the cafes or roof top gardens. I needed the fresh air, the natural light and thrived on breaking out of the endless restrictions I'd been adhering to for weeks now!

The days in that ward became some of the hardest and darkest for me. I started struggling on a few levels. The new medications really affected me, I was unable to sleep and even when I did, my dreams were so vivid I didn't realise I was sleeping, so tiring! Plus the meds made me ravenous, I was eating five full-sized meals a day to manage this crazy level of hunger. I could go from being perfectly rationale one moment to pure panic the next because I was so hungry.

However, the deepest concern was more subtle. I was basically the youngest, fittest, healthiest person on the neuro-ward; I felt so alone and misunderstood here.

I felt pure resentment and anger towards the hand I had been dealt, I cried tears into my mums' arms saying over and over again, 'this just isn't fair.' I became frustrated at everything. My independence had been so quickly replaced with being fully dependent on others in a matter of days. I couldn't shower myself, I couldn't go to the bathroom alone, I couldn't stand. I was stuck waiting and relying on other people to help me do anything and everything I needed.

One of the roughest nights was when a nurse burst in at midnight and told my mum she had to leave. Dad had taken mum's car home to be with my siblings so we looked back at her in confusion explaining she couldn't get home right then.

The nurse was irritated, *"Well you can't stay, visiting hours ended ages ago."*

Still puzzled I replied, *"I've had my parents staying with me every night since I got here; no one's said anything about it before."*

She stiffened, *"Why? We're being paid to look after you, you don't need them here. Or do you not trust us?"*

"It's not that. I just need my mum and dad here. I don't want to be alone here; everything I have gone through is so much – I just really need them." I started to sob.

"Jessica, everyone wants someone to stay with them I'm sure, but you're an adult. You need to get over yourself, you are being selfish stopping your parents from resting properly, they need rest so that they can look after you when you get home. We have social workers here if you need emotional support."

I just gaped up at her, "I don't want your social workers I just want my parents! Is that so hard to understand?"

She remained unmoved, "Your mother can stay here tonight, but I'm working tomorrow night and if she is here again after hours I will have her removed." With that threat she walked out.

This hospital just got worse and worse – I hated it and burst into tears again. Mum was angry at the way we had been spoken to and that night I didn't sleep. I didn't want to feel even more alone. All I wanted near me were the people who understood, the people I could rely on to talk to me when I couldn't sleep at 3am, the ones that would wipe away the tears and hold me tight while I cried about everything we had faced in the last ten days.

No woman with a clipboard, a degree and an attitude like that would understand what I was going through, what I needed. I felt pure hate for that nurse because she made me feel so small and so incredibly weak. It was a real knockdown when my strength and love of life were two things I was trying so hard to hang onto.

I felt cold and full of resentment, for the hospital, for the staff, I was done with this place. To my immense relief the doctors started talking about transferring me to a physical rehabilitation facility the very next day.

I still had to get through that night though and it was extremely tough, neither my parents nor I wanted me to be alone, but we knew that nurse was determined. It was horrible saying goodbye; I grabbed at their arms and held them tighter than ever.

I felt incredibly alone even though there were two other patients in my room with noises and nurses hopping around them. I felt empty. It dawned on me that my real fear of being alone related to the unwanted thoughts and emotions that rushed at me. I didn't want to feel the fear, the sadness, the anger, the frustration. I didn't want to contemplate the 'what ifs'. I wanted someone there to talk to, to take my mind off the shit and this truly awful situation. I was scared to admit to myself that what I was going through was so tough; it was honestly fucked. I liked pretending that everything was OK, that I was OK – because I didn't know how to cope if I wasn't OK.

I was livid when the nurse returned later that night with a smug look on her face.

"I'm glad you listened to me Jessica, I'm really proud of you for not being so selfish tonight."

It wasn't worth a reply.

I struggled through sleep that night, listening to music and watching movies; anything to avoid thinking and contemplation time.

After a restless night I woke up lethargic with headphones half in but at least the morning had come, I had survived my first night alone! I still couldn't wait for my parents to arrive. Thankfully they walked in just a few moments after I was told I'd be leaving soon for rehab. I happily assembled my things together so I could move on to my next adventure, one that I didn't fully understand yet.

As they rolled me out of the ward I remember thinking, 'thank goodness!' While Dr Marvel had been fantastic, and there had been some incredibly kind, caring and compassionate nurses and staff, there had also been many challenging and confronting experiences that shook me to my core.

See ya later gloomy rooms, I'm ready to walk.

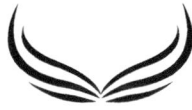

CHAPTER 8

STUCKNESS AND STARDOM

*"Do not judge me by my success, judge me by how many times
I fell down and got back up again."*
— *Nelson Mandela*

My parents and I played another exhausting game of 'wait for the transfer' before finding out I had to travel alone anyway and they'd have to drive. Everything took longer than expected so it was such a relief when I was eventually checked into my new private room at the rehab centre. Suddenly I found myself alone though, unsure what I was supposed to be doing. It was much quieter and slower paced here, it was strange just waiting for instructions from someone ... anyone?

My low FODMAP diet clearly perplexed the staff and a dietician came to see me first. I heard one of the nurses laughing, *"That's got to be made up!"* Not realising that I was already embarrassed by it enough as it was. It proved nearly impossible to find food in the hospital that I could eat; everything had onion, dairy or wheat, which were all hard no's for me. This created a lot of stress and anxiety, it may seem so trivial but my mind was blurry, I had an insane appetite and the thought of not having food sent me over the edge. My diet was literally the only thing I still felt like I had any form of control over in my life. The thought of losing the last shred of control was devastating, it made me feel helpless, needy and completely dependent, almost robotic, doing and eating what I was told, when I was told to. Thankfully within a day or two they had organised my own personal refrigerator for my room and made some special concessions for me.

My parents arrived bringing in the comfortable clothing I had requested and the right food to sustain me for the next day or two. Dad had his overnight bag in hand; we had readied ourselves for another battle to ensure someone was allowed to stay with me. After the anxiety and loneliness, I experienced on my one night alone at the last hospital, I knew I would need a familiar face around for my mental health and recovery. I was going to argue tooth and nail to have my way, so I went in nicely, asking, *"Is it at all possible to have one of my parents stay with me?"*

"Yes, absolutely," the head nurse replied. *"I'll organise a chair that can be converted into a bed at night and some sheets, however we cannot provide food for them."*

My jaw dropped along with my figurative fists and tears of gratitude filled my eye; he got it! No questions asked, he just got it and all I could manage to get out was an almost inaudible, *"Thank you."* It was so confusing that each hospital had their own set of rules I had to learn, I would have to advocate for myself at each step.

Although the head nurse was understanding, I still wasn't settled. I had so many changes to process; moving hospitals, the new environment, new nurse, new procedures; it was just another stack of changes to add to my already unbalanced and ever-growing pile to get used to. My life was beginning to feel like a game of Jenga; I didn't know which block would send me flying off the edge. The beauty was, no matter how many times my tower fell over I always found a way to rebuild it.

My first night in the hospital I was relieved to have my dad next to me. I barely slept five broken hours, mostly made up of lucid dreaming that I was in my bed awake! So exhausting! The most frustrating thing was waking up busting for the toilet only to have to wait 20 minutes before the nurse arrived to help me. I played videos, listened to sleep meditations, anything I could think of to get me to sleep. When morning rolled around I was awake and starving before the nurses or the food came around. I ate some of the snacks we'd hoarded in my drawers to get me through to breakfast time.

I asked to have an early shower, knowing I would need my nurse to help me the entire time. I understood why of course but that didn't make it easier. I felt so weak having someone else do everything for me. I stopped myself mid-pity party and reminded myself that this is what these beautiful nurses do every day. They help care for people who can't, they do it without shame, without complaining. They do it with compassion and in that moment my resentment for my situation was overrun by a humbling, heart-warming love for these incredible people and I was so grateful for them, because they could so easily be mean, resentful, uncaring and yet they're not. Whenever I felt resentment again, I tapped into this gratitude for them.

As the nurse helped me wash my hair, she was careful to avoid the staples that spanned more than 20cm in the middle of my skull from left to right. I still couldn't activate any muscles in my right leg so she held me up while I washed, giving me as much independence as I could manage. She made me feel human and that in itself was so beautiful, because I felt that I had lost all the things that made me 'me'; that made me an adult; that made me independent ... that made me worthy.

Despite being told that the doctors would come around after 9am, I was a bit baffled to see them walk in at 8.30am. I was alone; Dad had ducked out to find a good coffee while I was showering. I was torn between asking them to wait for him to come back because I knew how important it was to have a second set of ears in the room to help process the conversation. But I was also aware that I couldn't start physiotherapy until the doctors had cleared me. This really stressed me out. My entire purpose right then was to get back on my feet, to recover, to regain movement and get home as quickly as humanly possible. After wasting the day before and not seeing a doctor at all I didn't want to risk that happening again.

There were three doctors but one was clearly in charge with all the questions and answers, she was blunt and emotionless. Dr Blunt asked me how I was feeling.

"I'm pretty good given the circumstances," I answered with a smile, *"I've been struggling with sleep. I usually get 8 hours at home but at the moment I'm getting 4 or 5 but I know a lot of that is due to my body getting used to the new medications."* I sounded confident.

"OK, we can put you on an antidepressant." Dr Blunt was living up to her name.

My jaw dropped, *"I would hardly say I am depressed, I think my reaction to all the changes has been perfectly normal."*

Dr Blunt looked up at me as if I had insulted her, *"It will just help you sleep."*

I wished I had waited for Dad. I was becoming abrasive and stood my ground, *"I'm on enough medications as it is and I don't want to add another one unless it is necessary."*

She didn't look up from her clipboard. *"OK. What are your goals while you are here?"*

Phew! Back to talking about things that excited me like goal setting! I fired away.

"I need to learn to walk again and to get into my home, I need to be able to climb about 20 stairs." I said, the confidence and excitement of life back in my voice.

"And what do you plan on doing once you get out of here?"

I warmed to her again asking me about my aspirations. I hit her with my plans like a verbal bazooka.

"Once I'm off the steroids I can start my new life-saving treatment which we've been fundraising for. After I'm done with treatment I plan to go back to university and finish my final semester of my nutrition degree and then start my business and career as a motivational speaker!" This was the first time since I had been admitted that I had spoken so openly about what lay ahead once I was done with treatment.

The doctor looked at me like I was wasting her time, *"No, I mean what happens if you don't get better?"* Her tone was cold and emotionless. Her words burned like venom.

Tears threatened to pour out of my eye. *"I haven't entertained it; my brain surgery was successful and I am about to start on a treatment that will hopefully eradicate the disease."* I said with a plastered smile and snappy tone.

"With your condition, it's probably something you should be thinking about." She sassed back at me.

"Thanks for the advice but I CHOOSE to stay positive and focus on all the things I currently have working in my favour." I responded feeling jaded.

"Well if your current home can only be accessed by stairs and your cancer progresses then what?" She was a real piece of work. But I wasn't about to settle for her pessimistic outlook. Believing anything she said could be dangerous, or worse, a death sentence. I couldn't afford to think negatively. My life depended on it.

"Thanks for your concern but it's a rental property, I will deal with that scenario if and when it comes up and not a moment sooner. Now I'd appreciate it if you didn't talk to me like I'm on my death bed, this is my cancer, my diagnosis and my life. And I don't need you to make me more stressed than I already am. If you insist on being negative then I don't really want anything to do with you."

Dr Blunt had crossed a line of no return. She tried to pour her negativity all over me and I didn't want her toxic fumes. I didn't want other people's opinions, their facts, their concerns to impact my mindset. This was something I was extremely protective over, something that I worked at every day. Dr Blunt didn't speak to me again and I don't think I saw her after our first encounter. Perfect.

One of the other doctors had written my expected date to leave on my whiteboard, my heart sank to see it was three weeks away, a day after my treatment was meant to begin. I really did not want to be in hospital while I was going through treatment; I wanted to be in the comfort of my own home. When I mentioned that Dr Marvel had said I'd be here for two weeks at the most, the doctor was doubtful.

"We can assess you at two weeks but I don't believe you will be anywhere near ready to leave, you can't even walk and you need to be able to climb

20 stairs," said Dr Doubt.

Their business was over, and the doctors left just like that. They came in, spread their carnage and left me alone to pick up the pieces. I burst into tears, the confrontation with Dr Blunt shook me to my core, I felt helpless and alone and all I wanted to do was get out of this place. If I was well enough, I would have tied the bed sheets together and abseiled down the walls and out of the window like in the movies. Damn you cancer, right now I couldn't even walk.

~ Right in the Thick of It ~

Dad returned to see me in tears and just held me, telling me I was right to stand my ground. I refused to focus on what Dr Blunt had said and my mood lifted that afternoon when an OT came and organised my own personal wheelchair with a comfy seat and talked about joining the cooking classes and goals that excited me.

My first physio session was next, she had me up on my feet using the bed to balance, I was rather impressed with myself. When she told me to take a step, I looked at her in disbelief, how on earth would I do that? She encouraged me again and I thought I'd be smart by putting my functioning foot first. This inadvertently left me balancing on my uncoordinated right leg and I almost fell over. I wanted to laugh but I also felt a pang of fear. I would have to work so hard to even take five steps, let alone walk day to day, while running seemed out of the question! Little by little during that session, I made it around the bed as the beautiful physio helped me plant my foot correctly so I didn't stub, curl or hurt my foot. I left the physios room feeling excited, proud and absolutely exhausted but I knew that those few steps were just the beginning!

I had mixed feelings about the rehab centre, I loved the freedom that facility provided; spaced out nurse check-ups, outdoor areas and shared lounge rooms. I got permission to do physio sessions twice daily and had extra tasks to complete in between them. I could have free-flowing guests and on weekends I got to leave the hospital on day-leave. Dad took me out for walks pushing me around in my wheelchair. Or Mum would pick me up in her car and take me to a local café or to get my nails painted. I lived for the weekends when my friends could visit.

This freedom came with its challenges though, if I didn't have visitors I felt very isolated, there were less nurses which meant if I needed help getting to or from the bathroom. I could sometimes wait for 30 minutes or more, and often due to my lack of movement I was confined to my bed. The rehab centre was also close to a 90-minute drive from home which was exhausting for my parents and other visitors. I put in a request to be moved closer to home to lighten this burden, but it seemed to just get lost in the system. My mum ended up going back to work because of financial strain.

There were other young patients at the centre but many of them had acquired brain injuries and were being treated for both motor-neural and cognitive dysfunctions. One of the hardest things about this facility was that often the staff spoke to me like a five-year-old, looking back I understand why but at the time it frustrated me. I was cognitively functioning just perfectly; my only struggle was my lazy right leg. Even if I told them my cognition and understanding was fine, it usually didn't make a difference.

I also struggled to speak openly about having cancer. Being in a hospital for weeks on end made it so real and I couldn't talk about it without crying. I met some of the most beautiful and kind-hearted people in that facility, but I saw the sorrow and concern they had for me in their eyes. This would hit hard because I didn't want pitied looks, so I would shy away from interacting. I needed to be surrounded by people who made me feel normal, not like some poor cancer – riddled young woman who may not be around in three months. I wanted to laugh, to enjoy every day, to appreciate every moment I had on this earth.

Dad took me out one day for an appointment with Dr Energiser. We discussed increasing the rate I was weaning off steroids so I could start the dual immunotherapy sooner. I would have to return again for an information session about all the side effects and what to watch out for. I also had a check-up with Dr Marvel on my recovery from brain surgery. He was very excited to hear that I was walking even if it was extremely slowly.

Dad and I weren't due back at the rehab centre until much later so we ventured into the city. It was fun and exciting just doing normal things like buying new runners for rehab and stopping off at Zumbo cakes for a sneaky sweet treat. Being taken around in a wheelchair through Melbourne was a very sobering experience. Wheelchair access is limited in so many places and most people look at you as a burden. Especially on public transport, not wanting to make space or help my dad or me get on or off. During the lunch rush hour, people would often order or reach over me or cut me off like I didn't exist.

I have such a newfound respect for anyone who is wheelchair bound, it's far harder than it looks and it was a life-changing experience for me. The tramline back to rehab was supposed to be wheelchair accessible but when we got to our stop Dad had to lift me off in the wheel chair. Although there was a sea of young faces the only person who offered to help was a gentleman in his 60s! I was appalled at the lack of support and help offered, the dirty looks given for holding up people's day, but mostly I was appalled that I felt like a burden. After that I never wanted to get on public transport as long as I was wheelchair-bound or in a position where I might require help.

Dad was wonderful and would usually spend the nights with me. He'd take a break during the day, while Mum visited in the evenings. She would replenish my food stores and return my clean washing she'd done for me. When she tried to pack it away I told her no, because she didn't know where things went. I had gone from being relatively untidy to being obsessively organised, everything had its spot and I used to get very stressed if it wasn't in its correct spot. I could spend hours organising and reorganising things, because at this point it was one other thing I had control over so I took that control very seriously.

Once I was stable and improving steadily Dad took the opportunity to fly home to South Africa. He was having a lot of trouble with his business that urgently needed to be sorted and he wanted to be back in Australia before my first dose of treatment.

~ Better the Devil You Know ~

Every day I watched my body get stronger, my steps get longer and my ability to walk improve. After ten days of intensive physiotherapy I was able to climb stairs with the aid of a crutch and I could walk 60m in 6 minutes (with multiple rest stops). I was cleared by the doctors to start hydrotherapy too. My physio was really impressed and she thought I could be out a week earlier than expected! I was excited and Mum got things ready for me at home. However, the next day, a doctor said my transfer had been accepted and they were moving me to a centre closer to home that day.

I was confused, *"I don't want to go; my physio says I'll be ready to leave on Friday. It seems silly to move now."*

He was a bit annoyed, *"You said you wanted to move so we've organised it. If you don't go you will struggle to get into outpatient physiotherapy down there if you haven't been an inpatient. It could take weeks and undo all the work you have done, I would highly recommend you move."*

I was flabbergasted, *"I told you almost two weeks ago that I wanted to move, I've settled in here. What would be my other physio options?"*

"You'd have to travel up here twice a week."

I didn't know what to do, I didn't really have another option. This would be my fifth hospital in a month. I felt like a lost sheep being herded around without care or consent. I became distressed and overwhelmed with that gripping loss of control again. Why do they always make decisions without my consent? I had no choice, so I reluctantly agreed. When I explained to Mum over the phone she was irritated too. She had organised a meeting with one of her clients around the corner from me that day and she didn't understand the point of the move either.

I had my final physio session, which turned out to be mostly paperwork preparing for the move. I was sad to be saying goodbye as I had loved working with her. A nurse came in looking for me as I needed to be back in my room for final obs before I left. When the nurse saw my light bulb was flickering as we entered my room, she announced I couldn't go in as I was prone to seizures. She'd have to put me in the lounge and wait for the handyman.

"How long is that going to take? I have to pack right away to

be transferred!"

"*Shouldn't be more than an hour,*" she said with a smile.

My frustration rose, I wanted time to be ready to leave in an hour and this was pushing my anxiety levels over the edge.

"*Why don't you just turn off the light?*" I said.

She stopped right there. "*That's such a smart idea,*" and wheeled me back to my room. For goodness sake!

They seemed so adamant to get me out the door, luckily Mum walked in then and we spent fifteen minutes together rushing around and packing up before the transfer arrived. I didn't even get to go to the bathroom before we left. Mum stayed back to ensure we had packed everything and I was on my way to hospital number five in four weeks. The ride was long and every bump reminded me that I had an insanely full bladder.

This rehab centre was much older and darker than my last one. The paramedics said their goodbyes and handed over my paperwork. We waited a while before the check-in nurse took me over to a table in the lounge. She seemed disinterested as she completed a few forms and asked some questions.

"*How long do you plan on staying here?*"

Odd question, surely people don't plan to be in a physical rehab centre? I thought they stayed as long as the physios and doctors thought necessary and not a moment longer.

"*Not long, just until the weekend.*" My tone was optimistic.

She stopped writing, looked up at me in a temper. "*What do you mean?! You have to stay here for a minimum of two weeks or we don't get the proper funding from the government!*" She yelled as if this hospital change was my choice.

Stunned and overwhelmed, I just started crying. I already hated this place too! Maybe I just hated being an inpatient at hospitals.

"*Well it wasn't my choice, the doctor put in the referral. He said I had to come down here to be linked in properly to the outpatient services.*" I said between sobs.

"*Well you'll be here for two weeks.*"

I glared at her in outrage, "*You are not holding me hostage in here for longer than I need to be. I start my cancer treatment next week and I will not be in here when that starts!"* She looked at me like I was a child throwing a tantrum over nothing.

"You can explain that to the owner of this facility, they will not take too kindly to it." With that she stood up, *"I will find your nurse to take you to your room."*

She turned her back on me and walked away. I wanted to crawl up in a ball and cry. All I wanted was to be home in my own bed. I wanted to be here about as much as that grumpy lady wanted me here! I wiped away my tears when a nurse approached, I didn't want to be seen as weak or irrational. That wasn't me, my true personality is strong and bubbly but this whole situation made me feel quite the opposite.

They only had these old, rickety and oversized wheelchairs in stock which made wheeling myself around about ten times harder, the nurse ended up pushing me as we toured around. She listed the rules as she went, and boy, oh boy — there were loads of them! The freedom I'd gained from my last rehab centre was ripped away as she explained the dining rules, the physio rules, the sleep rules, the guest visiting-hour rules, going outdoors's rules, everything you can think of had rules! Annoying ones. Rules I wasn't too interested in following.

When she rolled me into my room I was surprised to see that I was back sharing a room. I had become used to the luxury of having a private room, and I was told that it wasn't something they did based on age. The nurse was lovely and wanted to help me with anything I needed but all I wanted was to be left alone, shut the curtains and allow me to cry my eyes out — which I did.

When Mum arrived afterwards with all the things I hadn't been able to transfer, I tried to show her around with pretend enthusiasm. But I felt beaten; this last move had taken it out of me. I felt all the walls caving in around me. An isolation like no other. After being yelled at by the woman signing me in, I couldn't keep my usual smile around and before long I was sobbing again. The hospital rotations had caught up with me. Dark clouds rolled into my soul and I felt like I was falling into a dark empty void. Depression began to knock at the doors of my mind and I was petrified that it was beginning to creep inside. Perhaps this darkness would overtake me entirely. I clawed through my mind for hope, for positivity, for anything that would prevent the dark monsters of depression to overtake my heart and mind.

Against my heavy feelings, I reached for something Granny had taught me when I was a child. Gratefulness. To find gratitude in everyday moments, no matter what. I began to scan the room for the small moments, the ones I'd normally look past as 'normal' and tried to see something beautiful.

Mum calmed me down and added some beauty of her own, *"It will be alright Jess, I know it's not ideal but you're so close to home and all your friends can come visit now."*

I heard a bell ring out, and a nurse popped her head in to say hurry along to dinner. She turned to mum and said, *"Sorry but there are no guests during meal times, you'll have to come back later."* I looked at her perplexed, I wasn't hungry, it was only 5.30pm and I really just wanted my mum, my safety blanket.

Mum began to push me but the nurse told her I had to do it myself. So I wheeled my massive, clunky wheelchair into the dining room and chose a table near the entrance because it was such a struggle. A staff member informed me that I wasn't allowed to have my wheelchair in the dining room, I would have to move to a normal chair. I sat there quietly with my head hung low, defeated. I felt so out of place and as the room filled up slowly with men and women who were all in their 70s and 80s. I just wanted to eat my food and get back to my room. But I couldn't move swiftly without my wheelchair.

A gentleman sat at my table, I tried to talk to him but he didn't really seem interested. Then another man joined us and they started talking like best friends and I felt like a ghost. Part of me wanted to leave the table, but when I looked around everyone seemed to be in their tight-knit groups. It was like I had slipped into an American high school from *The Mean Girls* movie. There were cliques everywhere; the jocks, the mathletes, the populars, the emos ... well maybe not eighty-year-old emos. But I felt like Lindsay Lohan in an aged-care facility and I wanted to go and eat my tray of food alone in the bathroom stall.

While I was zoned out, slowly eating the bland, tasteless hospital food a third man came in, he looked at me and said, *"You can't sit here, this is the boys' table."* The boy's table? This is worse than high school. Was this the Hollywood jock that ruled the rehab centre?

It hit harder than I ever thought. In one swift sentence this old man had just confirmed what I had been thinking all day; I don't fit in here. I felt helpless once again and tears streamed down my face.

Thankfully one of the nurses was watching and brought over my wheelchair so I could get out of the dining hall and into the lounge room, where I sat alone. I had hit rock bottom. I mean I was being bullied by people in their 80s! What had happened to my life?

The nurse made me a cup of tea and sat with me. *"Don't take it personally dear, they're worse than a group of high schoolers."* She said with a giggle, though I didn't find it very funny.

"I don't want to be forced to sit in there at meal times, I want to be able to share my meals with my family or my friends."

"Our rules work for the most part, a lot of the people here wouldn't have any human interaction if they didn't come out for meals, but I know you don't fit in to our usual patients and that needs to be accounted for. I am sure we can change the rules for you because we don't want you feeling more isolated by putting you in there." My heart filled with gratitude for her.

After that interaction I felt a little lighter, like someone was listening rather than just lumping me in with a group of people who were fifty years my senior and had completely different wants and needs. Not to mention well-honed bullying tactics. That night I had my mum and a few friends drop in, being close to home was a great bonus and just what I needed to keep the darkness at bay. I was finding some small things to feel grateful for.

When I made it back to my room, my gratitude-filled mind was set on making a conscious effort with the older woman I was sharing with, her husband was there too. They made such a beautiful couple and shared such love for each other and for life, they were in their 80s and had spent more than sixty years together! I was in true awe of their love. They also showed me such compassion and for the first time that day, I felt like I could make a connection with some of the people here, they weren't all going to make me feel like the odd one out.

That night I called Dad and recounted my day and the crap I had endured, the emotions flooded in and I was crying on the phone.

"I hate it here, I really do. I'm so young, I'm so out of place!"

After I'd let it all out. I started to feel bad that my lovely roommate, Margaret had heard everything; how I hated it, how I was the youngest by fifty years. I liked Margaret, and I wanted to keep making an effort with her, that I wasn't just putting on a façade of pleasantries.

When I opened my curtain, she could see I had been crying again, and she just smiled softly. We began talking away as if nothing had happened, like we were old friends. I heard all about her life and her family. She was kind and gentle and a strong Christian woman. She reminded me so much of my granny and that's why I felt so at home in our room. I opened up to her too. I shared my experiences, my diagnosis, the many moves. She saw me cry but this time it was in a beautiful way, I was connecting with her, I was being vulnerable and allowing her to see the real me. The one she'd heard behind the curtain, the young woman who was scared and vulnerable, who felt isolated and pushed around, the one whose life was filled with an overwhelming amount of uncertainty. But who was also grateful for every single day, a woman who smiled and found joy everywhere. A woman who had discovered the power of gratitude was helping her keep the darkness at bay.

When I reflected back, Granny had always taught me to be grateful, to count my blessings no matter what. The hospital marathon-moves had sent me into a dark downward spiral and without the lessons I now call 'Granny's Gratitude' — my life would not be the same. Gratitude was the number one thing that helped me climb out the darkness and embrace every day.

Hearing the bell ring the next morning, I was filled with new hope as I slowly walked down to breakfast, leaving my wheelchair behind. The nurses weren't too happy with my decision to walk unassisted and without their permission but too bad for them. I'd decided not to be the first in the dining room! Last night had taught me that I should chose my seat more carefully because apparently there are special spots. I must have looked like a deer in headlights as I scanned the room looking for a safe place to sit. A lively woman saw me and called me over as if we'd been friends for years! As I walked slowly over, I let go the breath I had been holding and sat down amongst this much more open, kind and welcoming group. I felt much happier. I was in their grey-haired clique. They made my gratitude list that night.

~ Holding Me Back ~

Although this centre was a lot closer to home, most of my friends worked or studied during the week so I spent a lot of the time just in my room with Margaret. It was very slow paced with not a lot to do. I was going a little stir-crazy being stuck inside and not exercising. A few professionals came in to do some basic evaluations and even my first physio appointment was frustratingly just a group of tests, very similar to the exit tests I had done before leaving the last facility.

I returned to my room feeling that I had taken a step back and lost two days of therapy which drove me mad! I felt like this whole place had set me back a lot. I would only get one physio appointment a day and I couldn't get into hydrotherapy without medical clearance. While I was feeling more comfortable with the people around me, I really struggled with this rehab centre, it just was not the right fit for me.

I really struggled with not being allowed to leave the building. I love being outdoors and the fact that I could not even go outside for a bit of fresh air was giving me cabin fever. I understood their reasoning; they didn't want patients to run off but as I wasn't able to run yet I figured I was a safe-bet and I desperately needed this outlet to keep me sane! After a lot of shameless pleading, one of the nurses opened a side door for me and allowed me to sit outside with a book and relax, that made my day! My gratitude list was growing.

I had an early physio session the next morning, and I asked if there was any chance I could do more. They said no but they had booked me in for hydrotherapy the following day, they were just waiting on the doctor's clearance. I was quietly confident knowing that I had been cleared at my last rehab centre. I kept doing as many exercises as I could in my room to keep my momentum going.

I wolfed down breakfast the next day, eager to go back to my room and change for hydro. Think kid at Disneyland level of excitement! It was in hospital that I really started to appreciate things that I had taken for granted; swimming, the outdoors, alone time and my independence. I listened for the knock that meant someone from staff was coming to move me. When it hit 7.55 I couldn't wait and pressed for my nurse. One of the student physio's I had met the day before popped in instead but she didn't seem in a rush to get me to the pool, obviously she didn't realise how much I wanted to be there.

"Shouldn't we get a wriggle on, it's a bit late." I said with an impatient but playful smile. I liked having a younger physio, someone in their 20s someone I could relate to.

"Unfortunately, the doctors won't give you clearance because you've had a seizure," she said with certainty.

"What do you mean? I've already been cleared at the last facility so why would they not give me clearance here? This is a joke! This place is literally just setting me back in my recovery!" I yelled with tears rolling down my face.

She stammered a reply then just when she looked like she was about to leave, I exploded!

"I hate this place. I hate everything about it. I'm just a number, I don't matter! My recovery and my mental health don't matter as long as my bed is filled for two weeks and I'm paying the bills – it doesn't matter! I just want to go home. I feel stuck and trapped here, instead of getting stronger, I'm getting weaker! I was doing two physio sessions a day at my last rehab centre and now I'm just wasting away here. I was meant to be going home this weekend and I don't see why I can't! I'm wasting valuable time here. I hate it and although this has been a tough month my mental health has not been as bad as it is in here. I'm lonely. I'm being bullied. I just want to go home!"

I ranted through sobs and tears. All the feelings from four challenging days here came to the surface and I could no longer contain my disappointment, my irritation and my anger at the situation.

I had tried to be understanding. I had tried to stay calm, to please others, to be polite but I couldn't do it anymore.

"*I just hate it here.*" I whimpered.

Looking up at the physio, she looked like she had never encountered such rage in her life, and my heart softened. While I hated this whole thing, I also hated the way I was behaving in that moment – it wasn't me at all.

"*I'm sorry, I know this isn't your fault,*" I said. "*It's too much for me, I've been in hospital for over a month and I'm missing my home and scared about starting treatment next week.*"

She still looked overwhelmed, but had compassion in her eyes.

"*I'll see what I can do.*" And she walked out.

I felt horrible and incredibly guilty. I tried to validate my actions and behaviours by telling myself it was good she was exposed to the frustration of her patients' feelings. But I couldn't shake my regret. I was glad I had got my feelings off my chest but not in that way, not at all! To my surprise, forty minutes later, the same young physio was at my door with a bright smile.

"*If you can get ready we will put you in for another physio session this morning.*"

I beamed at her, "*Give me two minutes!*"

Relief flowed through me for two reasons; first that I hadn't impacted this young physio's day or caused her to quit! And also because I was getting to move my body! We chatted together, me apologising profusely for the way I had behaved, and then I found out it was her birthday! Oh crap – I felt so bad! We set to work for over an hour that morning, another young student physio joined us as well. I felt so much better and was excited to know I had another session that afternoon.

Later that day, a doctor came in to tell me they had decided to move forward my discharge to the following day and I was overwhelmed with joy. I cried for a second time that day but they were tears of happiness. I knew that part of this had happened because of my little breakdown earlier. I felt bad that the physio had taken the brunt of it, but seeing the outcome, that the ball was finally rolling and I was getting out of here. This made me so incredibly happy that I was glad that I'd spoken up. I quickly called Mum to share the news.

The change in plan caused a large influx of professionals to walk into my room to talk logistics, do tests, work out what I would need to rent out and take home with me, things like shower seats and special chairs. My final physio appointment was an assessment to tick-off everything and get on my way.

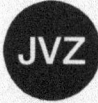

JVZ **Jessica Van Zeil** •••
My Facebook post from that day

After 1 month, 5 hospitals and countless goals achieved I finally got the all clear to go home tomorrow.
This month has challenged me more than I ever anticipated. There have been tears, frustration and absolute exhaustion. But also, excitement, passion and gratitude beyond belief. I am so proud of the person I am and how I have gotten through this.
Watching my body change and get through this bump in the road has been incredible. I have been getting stronger every day and making huge strides. I have never been more in love with my body. It's taken a huge knock from being a fit, healthy 23-year-old to being in bed and hardly able to move for the first few weeks. I have had huge changes to my diet and a million medications pumped through me but I got through this. #happyandhome

That evening, I shared the news with Margaret and her husband, they prayed for me and wished me well for my next challenges as I would start immunotherapy soon after getting home. I was sad to say goodbye to the woman who was my saving grace in that place. I walked in excitedly telling anyone who would listen that I would finally be home tomorrow and get to see my dog!

I was already packed and ready to go when Mum arrived the next morning!

Getting home was daunting when I looked up at the stairs; it took me ten minutes to climb them. I was exhausted by the top but so incredibly grateful to be home, to relax, to be in my own space. However, we had to make some adjustments. I moved into Mum's room so I was close to the bathroom and I would still need her help to shower. I realised my wheelchair was not ideal in the house, I was better off walking slowly than trying to manoeuvre around the small spaces at home.

Coming home from rehab made me feel accomplished, I'd finished that chapter in my life and I was ready for the next. That confidence made me feel invincible, and I pushed myself far harder than I needed to. I didn't want to rest; I had spent the last month doing that. I wanted to move around the house, pottering, helping, cooking and creating. This urge to be doing things knocked me down though, I would push myself to the brink and then require a three-hour nap. I was completely off the steroids which had helped keep me wired and awake for weeks — but now my body craved all the hours of sleep I'd missed while on the super 'roids.

I still insisted on getting out of the house though, I was sick of feeling trapped in a prison of protection. I had so much I wanted and needed to get done. The second day home I had a mini meltdown. I had a massive interview coming up with 60 Minutes for a segment on Youth Cancer. I had given a speech when the Youth Cancer Centre opened and they had approached me to do a media piece about it.

My clothes either didn't fit anymore or weren't easy enough to put on and be comfortable enough to sit in all day. I went shopping with Mum and found myself frustrated and irritable, the fluorescent lights gave me migraines and made me feel sick, this was a new discovery and probably a result of the seizure. Getting in and out of changerooms, finding clothes to fit; it was all so much harder than I had expected.

The other mission occupying my mind was that our fundraising page for my dual treatment would finally be released on the same day as the interview. What an epic day! My family and I had put so much work into it for so many weeks, I was anxious for it to go well. There had been so much change and turmoil to process in just a few days, no wonder I was feeling overwhelmed. But I had discovered something amongst the turmoil. That gratitude can keep someone sane.

That just seeing a sunset or the sunrise from my room could change the dark moment if you look for it. No matter how difficult the news was, no matter how many intense emotions I went through finding something beautiful to focus on and be grateful for made my time in hospital easier. It literally was the essential that saved me from slipping into that deep dark hole of depression.

Chuffed.org – Fundraiser Launch

Help a fighter keep fighting against cancer

If you need proof that Jess is a fighter, you won't need to dig too deeply. At just 22, she made the toughest call, to have her left eye completely removed. Jess is a powerfully positive and ridiculously resilient girl and there is no one better suited to beat this rare and aggressive form of cancer, ocular melanoma.

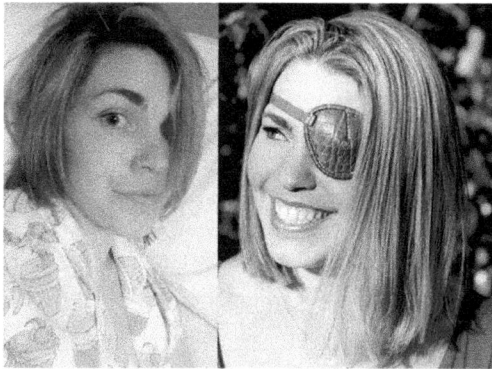

Her strength to confront a decision like this and her resolve in the months afterwards, proves she's someone who will never back down from a challenge no matter how difficult it may be. If you asked her, she'd tell you that she has an extraordinary support group and a fantastic family who helped her cope through these tough times. The truth is though; mostly she's done it herself. She has bravely dealt with adapting to life with an eyepatch, confronted by her present and redefining her future. Even in imagining the future, she has been

powerfully positive and selfless, hoping to use her story to inspire and help others.

Jess now needs your help! Four weeks ago, Jess had a seizure, out of the blue, and in hospital we were told she had tumours in her brain. The cancer has seeded itself and there are at least four areas of concern in her brain. Jess' cancer is very difficult to treat and the only option, which could help her survive, is a new immunotherapy treatment. Unfortunately, the cost of this medication is over $100,000, far beyond what our family can afford. The treatment needs to start immediately to give Jess the greatest chance of winning this fight. As a family, we hate to ask for help, but nothing is more important to us than doing whatever it takes to give Jess the best hope of beating this terrible disease.

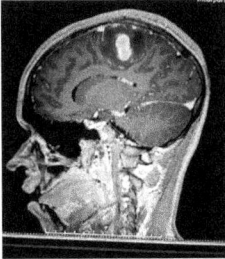

Surgery was required to remove a 3cm tumour and leaves our beautiful Jess unable to walk on her own. Unfortunately, this type of cancer cannot be resolved by surgery alone.

She has many tough days ahead of her, even with the treatment. Already determined to re-learn how to walk, she'll now likely have to cope with sickening side effects of this medication. It will hurt us to watch our active and passionate girl have to go through that but it will be worthwhile.

If you would be willing to help via a donation on this site, Jess, her family and friends will be eternally grateful. You'll be helping a born fighter keep fighting and she will not let you down if given the chance. **Please make a donation now by clicking on the right of this page.**

Some questions you might have.

What is the treatment my donation will fund?

You will help Jess to receive a new immunotherapy treatment and cover both the drugs themselves and her ongoing treatment. Delivered over 4 treatments, a blend of two drugs called Opdivo and Yervoy will be administered. This treatment literally teaches Jess' immune system to target and fight the Melanoma cells.

What are the chances of the treatment working?

This treatment is so new that Jess will be one of the first to use this combination of drugs on Metastatic Melanoma on the Brain. The combination of Opdivo and Yervoy has shown promising results with other, similarly difficult to treat cancers and there is quite a lot of info online about them.

How much should I donate?

Anything you can contribute will make a difference! Our family is extremely grateful. Thank you for helping our Jess in the biggest fight of her life.

Does all that I donate go to Jess' treatment?

100% of the funds raised on Chuffed.org go directly to Jess' treatment. The site does not take a cut, instead, they ask for a voluntary contribution to them. This is entirely at your discretion.

How else can I help?

If you would share this page either directly to your friends and contacts or on your own social pages, and ask others to support Jess, it would be a massive help.

Where can I learn more about Jess and her story?

Jess has her heart set on using her story to inspire others through a career in public speaking. Check out her website www.jessvanzeil.com

How can I keep track of Jess' progress?

Jess will soon be adding a blog to her website and plans to write fortnightly. You'll soon also be able to register to receive updates via her newsletter. Also, if you want to you can follow Jess on Instagram @Jessvanzeil

How do I know this is legit?

Jess has been very vocal and public in supporting the Victorian Government and Peter Mac in raising awareness of the needs of young cancer patients. You can see details through a web search of her name or visit this link – Peter Mac.

Earlier this year Jess was very involved with the Melbourne Melanoma March, she spoke at the event and later held her own fundraiser to help raise money for Melanoma research.

On Jess' website, there will be video and other updates of her treatment and progress. The treatment Jess needs is easily researched online.

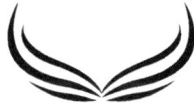

CHAPTER 9

DUAL TREATMENT:
GETTING SICK MEANS GETTING WELL?

"To conquer frustration, one must remain intensely focused on the outcome, not the obstacles."

— *T.F. Hodge*

I was excited that Dad was returning from South Africa in time for my first treatment. After he landed, he met Mum and I at the Youth Cancer Centre where we would be interviewed by Peter Overton from 60 Minutes.

Mum, Dad and I sat huddled around the laptop beforehand, coffee in hand as we nervously went live, praying that with the help of my peers we would manage to reach our goal. Within minutes of posting it we saw the donations flowing in, but we had to get back to the interview.

As I was preparing my make-up before the interview, I looked in the mirror but didn't recognise the girl looking back at me. I saw the effects of the steroids and other medications; from the puffy moon face, the pimply irritated skin, the limp right foot and the bony body that seemed so frail. My reflection didn't look like the strong Jess I knew, cancer had taken its toll on me and I felt self-conscious to be seen on TV this way.

However, when I looked deeper than these insecurities, I saw proof in these side-effects. Proof that I had chosen once again to fight for my life, no matter what the cost. They were evidence that I had walked through the depths of hell on earth and was still smiling. I was still winning my battle with cancer because no matter what I looked like, I was still *me* shining through. I was tough. I was smart. I was funny. I was happy. I was grateful. I was wise. I was beautiful. Maybe not in the way beauty is usually defined, it was far deeper than that, I had a light inside me that no one was putting out and as long as that light shinned in this interview, as long as they saw me for me, I was happy with that!

I loved the interview process, I felt so comfortable, like I was talking to a friend. I also found the 'industry tricks' interesting, like the retake from behind the head and counting to five to get the right angle in head movements. When the day ended, we had over two hours of footage; I was exhausted but so proud. I smiled and laughed, I spoke my truth, I was me and I felt beautiful. I fell asleep on the drive home and needed to rest and take it easy.

Much to my mum's dismay the next day I wanted to head out on another adventure. It was great having Dad to hang out with, while everyone else still had their study and working lives during the week Dad wheeled me around Mornington as we explored shops, visited friends and drank coffee. Although it was a far stretch from my normal life, I was so grateful just to be able to get out and do or see things I had missed in my hometown. I was also celebrating the fact that we'd reached $30,000 on our fundraiser in 24 hours! Which was enough to cover the cost of my first dose of treatment. I was exhausted but it was so worth it.

Not knowing how long treatment would take, the next day I packed a few books, my laptop and headphones before heading off to the hospital. Before it started, I was told about all the potential side-effects; I wasn't going to lose my hair or experience the usual nausea and vomiting associated with cancer treatments, however I could face liver failure, hormonal imbalances, bowel disease, vertigo and about thirty other scary things. I was given a list of symptoms and told to call my designated nurse, 'nurse angel', if I experienced any of them. If caught early they were treatable, if left too long they may cause long term side-effects and maybe even result in death. Ironically, the treatment that was my best chance at surviving could also cause my death. If the moment wasn't so shocking I could have laughed out loud from the ridiculous irony.

The treatment works by building up your immune system, however when your immune system is too strong it can start to attack healthy cells, like an autoimmune disease. The most ludicrous part of all was that the worse and more prevalent the side-effects were, the more likely it was to have a positive effect shrinking the tumour. In a nutshell, the sicker I could be, the better. An odd paradox to feel good about.

Initially I was grateful that I wouldn't lose my hair, however this became something I almost resented. I didn't look 'sick enough' or have the typical chemo side-effects so I was seen as 'lucky', but my hidden side-effects were just as scary and life-threatening.

It was a strange situation to be in. Battling a disease that was desperately trying to kill me and yet not looking 'sick enough' to fit the stereotype. I was often told by others that I didn't look like I had cancer. Sometimes it felt like a weird and distorted type of discrimination — not gaunt enough or hairless enough to be considered unwell but still fighting for my life.

The chemo ward was huge, I lost count of the rooms as I was wheeled through to my chemo seat. My room had six other seats each filled with a person who had a drip pumping some magical medication into them that they hoped would save their lives. Some slept, some had people surrounding them, others had laptops or a book in hand. I sat nervously with my parents on either side wondering what came next. We got a bit restless as it took almost two hours for the treatment to be prepared. Later we understood that because my treatment was so costly they didn't prepare it until I was actually sitting on the ward, then the preparation on its own took an hour minimum.

Luckily, for my parents, since my steroids had dropped my raging hunger had died down dramatically. No more was I like a toddler in their terrible twos throwing a tantrum over the wrong flavour of milkshake, which was probably the right flavour when it was ordered.

I could sit through the whole regime to administer it without being hangry — (hungry and angry at the same time). The first bag was given over two-and-a-half hours, then there had to be a ninety-minute gap before the next treatment which took another ninety minutes, and then flushing and observations for another hour. By the time my treatment was done I was the last person in the room and probably the whole ward, it was 8.30pm. By this stage, I was tired, hungry and grumpy as we still had the hour-long drive home.

The next few days I was exhausted, bed-ridden and headachy. These were things I was told to expect and hoped would pass. However, on the fourth day after treatment, I woke up at 5.30am with a debilitating headache. I was in the most intense and crippling pain, I stumbled to the bathroom and started throwing up, Mum held back my hair; I could feel her panic. The headache was so bad I physically couldn't walk or open my eye; the sunshine felt like fire as it hit my eye, I needed a pitch-black room. Even the heavy-duty pain medication Dad brought around didn't help. Mum made numerous calls to the Peter Mac Cancer Centre and eventually we were advised to head into the our local hospital. Mum could see the massive pain I was in and how incredibly weak and unstable I was so she called an ambulance; my 8-day hospital breakout was over.

The paramedics quickly realised I couldn't speak beyond a mumble or a groan and that I had the same adversity to the sun as a vampire. Once at the hospital I was placed in the hallway as there were no beds available. I was given a magical non-vomiting pill – seriously they are incredible and whoever invented them should be given a Nobel prize — the nausea and vomiting eradicated within minutes. The emergency room was loud and bright, I tried to sleep to get some relief but being stuck in the hallway was rather unnerving. I was so lucky that a beautiful nurse and family friend happened to walk past me in the hallway and promptly organised a room that was out of the way.

We waited an eternity. Other than a quick CT scan I wasn't seen by a doctor for eight hours! I was on edge and although I was in pain I was also terrified that my cancer might be progressing or another tumour had haemorrhaged; the waiting just gave me extra time to stress and worry. Eventually when the doctor arrived, I could still barely open my eyes. *"So, you're here for a headache?"* he said looking down at his sheet with an unimpressed tone.

What! Had he not read my file? The headache may be a symptom of something far more sinister. I grimaced through the excruciating pain to let Dr Dismissive know the deal.

"Not just any headache. I'm in a ridiculous level of pain and have been since this morning, followed by vomiting. I'm worried it's a side-effect of the cancer progressing or the new treatment I'm on, so no, it's not just a headache!" I sassed back at him, my parents looked just as disgruntled.

"Well it doesn't look like anything so I'm going to send you home tonight."

My eye nearly popped out of my face and my voice rose in panic.

"Firstly, have you got clearance from my team at Peter Mac Cancer Centre to send me home? Without that I am not leaving. Secondly, there are twenty steep steps to climb up when I get home and I'm recovering from brain surgery and have only just relearned to walk this month, I don't feel safe going home, that's why Mum sent me in an ambulance this morning!"

He just looked at me with an air of irritation, *"Why didn't you mention the stairs before?! Now I'll have to find you another bed."*

I stared in disbelief. Dr Dismissive didn't think stage 4 cancer, the new treatment or even the blinding headaches were of any concern, but the stairs? God forbid, we had stairs! And they were the reason he would keep me in!

I was moved into an overnight bed in the emergency department. But after my interaction with Dr Dismissive, I felt out of place and like I was overreacting; even though I was in agony, strangely, I somehow felt like wrong for being there.

The next morning, I woke up to a smiling older doctor, Dr Smiles was intrigued by my case as he was one of the hospital's oncologists. I felt calmer when he reiterated that I had done the right thing by coming in. He wanted to get in touch with Dr Energiser and organise for me to be transferred to my treating hospital that afternoon.

Once I was transferred, the doctors ran a battery of tests from scans to bloods but after almost a week of being trapped in another facility I was sent home. The funny thing was that I wasn't itching to get out like before. I was really hoping for an answer, coming home without any explanation of what happened was hard. I was told that it was likely to just be my body reacting to having a multitude of new medications introduced and taken away over the last month. Thankfully they decided to continue on with treatment despite this little hiccup.

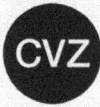

CVZ

Craig Van Zeil is with **Jessica Van Zeil**
18 October 2016 ● ● ●

Hi, it's been a while since I have given you all an update, I just thought that everyone needed a bit of a break in Jess news.

I heard a whole lot of people had put in a request for the name of Facebook to be changed to Jessbook, as everyone's walls were just full of Jess postings and re-posts :)

As you know Jess had her infusion drip last week Wed. She was pretty buggered Thurs, Fri and Sat and then suddenly on Sunday she got hit with chronic headaches. I had her rushed to hospital and she has been admitted to try and work out what is happening

It might be a side effect but they just don't know. So, they are doing test by test to eliminate all other options and hopefully we will have an answer in a day or so.

So back in hospital for Jess! I guess it is the reality of cancer that we all have to get used to. Every day is a new day and we just take it as it comes.

I have attached a few pics of Jess in hospital. Today we went out for coffee, wheel chair, drip machine and all. I often wonder what people must think of us! But we were getting out there no matter what!

The good news is that Jess's fundraiser broke $50k today. It sounds like a fortune and I guess it is, but we are not even halfway there.

We wanted 13,000 people to donate $10 and relatively 5000 people's worth of $10 has come in.

We are so appreciative of all your efforts already and remember please tell your friends, because every bit counts and what is $10 today anyway when it can go to save a young girl's life?

Lots of love xx

~ Living in Limbo ~

It was a hard time after I returned home again. The excitement of being back in my home territory had lessened, the university exam period had started and Dad had left for South Africa again. I felt even more alone, less people visited and Mum was back at work. My siblings didn't seem to understand that while I was home I was still a long way from a full recovery and very much dependant on the people around me. My rigid obsession with cleanliness that had started in hospital grew. I kept my room immaculate, I freaked out if the kitchen was untidy and I pushed myself to exhaustion as I tried to fix these things and do my laundry and maintain my fitness and recovery. There were days where I insisted on doing my washing but after hanging my stuff on the line, I was so exhausted I had to nap for two hours!

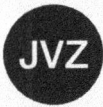

JVZ **Jessica Van Zeil** •••
27 October 2016

Frustration is an overwhelming emotion that I have had a few run-ins with lately.

6 weeks ago, I went from complete independence to complete dependence and while I'm slowly getting back some of my mobility and independence I have a long road ahead of me.

Sometimes everything becomes a little too much. I get caught in the stress of the moment, I forget to breathe and just appreciate every

day. It's these moments when it's important to remember to embrace
every challenge because it's these challenges that help us grow.

The three weeks between treatments rolled around quickly
and it was time for my second dose of treatment; we requested
an earlier time slot remembering how long it took first time
around. There was also a film crew there to record extra shots for
my 60 Minutes interview. I showed off my mad walking skills; a
whole 50 metres just for them! I was exhausted after that walk
but I impressed even myself. They took various shots of me in the
wheelchair, then of Mum, Amy and I in the chemo ward talking and
hanging out while I had treatment.

After the crew left, we still had endless hours of waiting and
being pumped with my lifesaving meds. Even though we started
earlier we were still the last people on the ward. I sleepily walked to
the car, knowing this time I needed to allow myself to rest. I spent the
first two days after treatment in bed, resting, reading and relaxing.
As the days went on I regained my energy and was able to do more
and more, although I still required a nap every day.

Ten days after my second dose, I was due for my first set of
scans since being diagnosed with stage 4 Melanoma, although at
that point I refused to admit that I was stage 4; it was simply
terrifying. I knew these scans were incredibly important, they were
an indicator as to whether the treatment was working. There were
three outcomes all as likely as each other. One, they had grown.
Two, they had shrunk and three, they were the same.

I was filled with *scanxiety* (a scan-related anxiety, a phenomenon
that most cancer patients experience in the days and weeks leading
up to their scans).

Logically I knew it wasn't the scan's fault if there was a change.
Even if I didn't have the scan done it wouldn't change what was
happening inside my body. I was stuck between the fear of not
knowing and the fear of knowing. The scans were like a great

unmasking. What if the results were bad, did I really want to know that? Especially after all the effort we put into getting me this far.

My life was once again dangling off the edge of a cliff and the rope could snap at any moment, or it could stay strong? There were no guarantees either way.

Any lies I had been telling myself or had believed about myself and my body were going to be revealed. There was no hiding from the result. But even if the results were good there were no guarantees they'd stay that way. Limbo land was a frightening place to be.

Usually I would keep myself busy in the lead up to scans but this time because I was still so exhausted and physically drained I couldn't use my old coping mechanisms. I had to sit in my fears and face the barrage of emotions and my mortality head on. There was no hiding this time and that was tough.

In some ways it was good, it was the first time I allowed myself to really feel the emotional turmoil, the anger, the fear, the sadness. But it also brought in gratitude and joy unexpectedly, it made me realise how amazing every day was, it made me grateful that I had given myself the best shot by taking on this treatment, I understood nobody's days are a given and I was going to do everything, every single day to make my chances better, stressing wasn't worth it. While I was extremely scared I couldn't let it takeover my life for the next week, after all I thought, *"What if this week is my last?"*

The results were neither good nor bad, they were stable.

Stable was perhaps something I should have celebrated but it felt anticlimactic. I had no indication if the treatment was working or not. I knew nothing more than I had going in and it was weird. We were trying to shoot a target in pitch-black, we had no clue if we were aiming in the right direction so we just had to keep pulling the trigger hoping we were on the right track. These feelings only unsettled me more, I felt ungrateful. Although I hadn't gone backwards, I was in limbo and at the drop of a hat I could move backwards. I had no security and so I grieved for the outcome I had been hoping for.

Luckily, I had practiced looking for gratitude each day when I was in hospital, soon enough I came to see that being stable was great. I was eight weeks post seizure and there had been no change, my initial tumours had grown in a four-month period and they were now stopped in their tracks. Whether it was just buying me time or meant I was on the road to recovery was irrelevant because right in that moment I had days ahead of me and that was enough! A warrior-like energy of living for now, living in the present filled me.

The three weeks between each treatment were much the same. I had treatment mid-week, which left me tired, headachy, and requiring bed rest for the next three days. By the Sunday I felt well enough for something exciting and social like brunch or a trip to the local craft market. Then on the Monday I would have a check-up with Dr Energiser. I made the most of the rest of my time by doing group physiotherapy three times a week; I was driven to recover as quickly as possible as my dreams were waiting for me. I knew I'd have to take care of myself as my exercise levels increased.

I was focusing so hard because I was 100% determined to still go on my trip to New Zealand to hike the Milford Sound in March 2017. My best friend and I had booked it well before my seizure. I knew that with hard work and strength building it would still be possible to conquer this hike. I shared this goal with the physio at one of my first sessions with him. He smiled at the excitement in my voice, and led me out into the long hallway and simply said, *"Well, let's get started."* I looked at him puzzled. *"What are you waiting for? It's your time to run."*

My mouth went dry and I stammered in fear, *"I ... I ... what do you mean? I don't know how to run."* The 15-metre hallway may as well have been 1000 kilometres; in my mind it looked impossible.

He laughed kindly, *"Didn't you say you used to love running?"*

My brow furrowed, *"Yes ... but everything's changed, my body doesn't respond like it used to. What if I land wrong and hurt myself or I fall. I just can't."*

He smiled again, *"Of course you can and I'll help you!"* He looped his arm through mine and lifted it up to stabilise me. *"OK, now go."*

I felt my hand get sweaty, I was terrified; I didn't know how to even start. I leapt forward feeling off balance and wobbly but the physio's arm held me straight. I gained momentum and although I felt like I looked like a (wo)man trying to walk on the moon I got to the end of the hall and tears filled my eyes. I had done it!

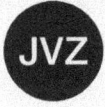

Jessica Van Zeil is at **Oliver's Hill**
30 November 2016   •••

What a crazy week! From treatment last Wednesday to increased physio load and starting a new training regime that actually has me running – I'm nowhere near ready to run a marathon but 30m is a good start.

With all this extra work and the stress of upcoming scans I have been feeling weak and exhausted. It's times like these when it's important to reflect, not on how I was going before my seizure but at how far I have come in less than 3 months! On the 16th of September I woke up from a surgery not knowing if I would ever walk again, with persistence, hard work and a lot of help from my family, friends and the incredible health professionals I deal with on a weekly basis my hopes of being able to run, hike and become completely independent again are finally looking achievable.

I never knew how strong I was until I was pushed so far out of my comfort zone it seemed "normal" was impossible. Instead of giving up I created a life outside of my comfort zone that challenges me daily, sometimes more than I would like to admit! It's been a rewarding journey that has made me appreciate my life and everyone/everything in it".

On December 14 2016, I had my final dose. I had been incredibly blessed that aside from a few headaches and dizzy spells I had avoided any major side effects. Added to this blessing was having all the money for treatment fundraised!

When I met with Dr Energiser after my final dual treatment, the first thing he said was, "*Congratulations! Thanks to you, sixty-six people in this hospital alone have started the dual treatment, a treatment many of them could not have afforded if it was not on the PBS."*

My eye welled up with tears realising for the first time that everything I had been through, all the videos and exhausting hours of campaigning to pay for my treatment had paid off a million times over – we hadn't just saved my life but this could save thousands of other Australians! It finally felt like my struggles had a bigger purpose. I knew that my age and special case was a driving force behind my fundraising being so successful. People were more generous when they heard my age and my story, I reminded them of their daughters, their nieces, they saw I had my whole life ahead of me if I could get treatment and they wanted to help me. I couldn't have been more grateful.

I had been able to use social media to my advantage, to help me raise the awareness by sharing my story, which helped us gain momentum in our goal to get my treatment onto the PBS. It was also a platform I could use to say thank you. (From the bottom of my heart a massive thank you to everyone who helped me fundraise and get treatment. Without your support, I may not have been here but more importantly hundreds if not thousands of other Australians would be unable to access this incredible treatment.)

Dr Energiser could see how moved I was by this news, he held the space for me and allowed me to experience the pure pride and joy that was overwhelming me.

Next, we discussed that in the New Year I would be starting two years of maintenance immunotherapy, it would be a single treatment once every 2 weeks, with less likelihood of any adverse side effects. He asked me what I had planned next in life and I spoke excitedly about the hike in New Zealand that I was still preparing for, and that I wanted to finish university before moving onto anything else. It was weird; finishing treatment had felt so far off, something that would never come. The future seemed scary and still filled with unknowns but I was excited to see one.

He asked if there were any changes he needed to know about and I mentioned that my GP had taken me off my contraceptive pill because it was clashing with another one of my medications. Dr Energiser cautioned me on two fronts, *"I must warn you, do not get pregnant while you are on this treatment, you would be risking your life."*

I laughed, *"Don't worry, I am completely and happily single with no men on the scene whatsoever, I've been slightly too preoccupied to date."*

It was funny discussing my single status with Dr Energiser so before I left his office he gave me some added advice about studying. He suggested I take a step back, reminding me I was still very unwell, much sicker than most people who defer, perhaps I should focus on getting better first.

It wasn't until later at home that I rehashed our conversation. I laughed again at the thought of getting pregnant; I thought it was lucky that I knew I didn't want my own babies, I wanted to adopt. But a little voice inside me wondered whether I'd feel like that forever or if my desires might change. It scared me a little because while I knew I wanted to adopt it had previously been a choice, an idea I had mulled over. Knowing that it may be my only option to have a family of my own, well that was scary. I put it to the side for the time being thinking, 'Let's just get through this cancer thing first, then we can think about kids. Or even going on a date for the matter.'

As for university, I thought long and hard about Dr Energiser's recommendations. I knew I was sick and exhausted, but I also really wanted it done. My thoughts by then were logical and clear in the face of my own mortality. I said to myself, 'If I don't make it past the next year I want to have finished the one thing I started in my adult life, I want my degree, even if I don't plan on using it. And if I do survive this, I don't want my study looming over my head.' I wanted my options open, my future bright.

> *We keep moving forward, opening new doors, and doing new things, because we're curious and curiosity keeps leading us down new paths.*
>
> — *Walt Disney*

Jess is sharing so much more in her INTERACTIVE book.
See exclusive, behind-the-scenes videos, audios and photos of Jess's journey.
DOWNLOAD free content and learn how to become powerfully positive and ridiculously resilient.
deanpublishing.com/eyewon

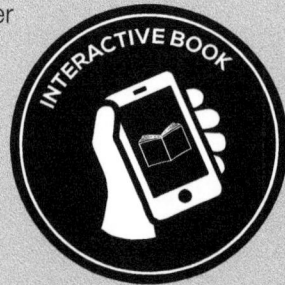

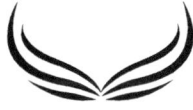

CHAPTER 10

AN UNUSUAL CHRISTMAS SPIN

*"The oak fought the wind and was broken, the willow
bent when it must and survived."*

— *Robert Jordan*

I was rapt to think my treatment and appointments were over for the year and I could finally focus on celebrating Christmas!

In the days leading up to Christmas, I was feeling really unwell, dizzy spells, exhaustion, stomach pains. None of it seemed particularly out of the ordinary or what I classed as ordinary, but I did feel off. It caused me to miss out on so much and I started to feel even more alone. Many people assumed now that treatment was over I was in the clear. So many times I was left home alone because I was too tired or sore to join them but I didn't want to complain and make other people miss out or worry about me.

I underplayed what was going on because I felt I was a burden, I was needy and I was ruining everyone else's fun. I tried to keep those feelings at bay, and celebrate the fact that I had made it to

Christmas – my favourite time of year. I celebrated with family, laughing, smiling and having fun. Dad had come over from South Africa for my final treatment and was staying in Melbourne. He came down to be a part of my mum's family Christmas. Although they weren't together, my family understood how important it was to me and the rest of my siblings to share this day with both of our parents.

On Christmas Eve, I managed to laugh and exchange some presents with my family but inside I started to panic at the feeling of nausea and dizziness creeping in. This was the last thing I wanted to put my family through with so much on over the next few days. Fortunately, it passed and I spent the evening with my beautiful family. Christmas morning was our traditional opening of Christmas stockings and then heading to church.

Afterwards things worsened at Granny's for lunch, the excitement of Christmas was too much for my body and I napped for hours on the couch, it was the only way to stop the room from spinning. Arriving back home, I took one look up at the stairs and started crying, going up them felt like a climb up Mt Everest. I finally confessed to Mum that I was feeling really horrible. She helped me inside to lay down and hopefully rest would help but the dizziness just got worse. To my disgust, there was no choice but to get back in the car and head back to the emergency department.

I had really wanted to avoid going to hospital at Christmas, I knew how busy it would be with lots of drunken antics and injuries due to fights. But by this time I had to, my dizziness was so bad I couldn't stand on my own, I was grabbing onto Mum as we patiently waited at triage. I was silent but the tears threatened to pour down my face as I panicked internally as to what all this could mean.

There was a large line for triage and I knew that everyone around me felt the same so we waited patiently. The guy behind me however believed that he shouldn't have to wait and kept grumbling under his breath, I did my best to ignore his incessant and derogatory comments. Eventually I was called to the front, I was extremely lucky to have a special card that got me to the front of the line and admitted almost immediately after a few questions; #cancerperks.

I explained to the triage nurse that I was extremely dizzy and faint, a possible side-effect of my dual immunotherapy treatment for Stage 4 melanoma, and that I was recovering from brain surgery. She swiftly moved me to the final check-in station, she could see my fears and that I was biting back my tears.

"Don't worry we'll have a bed for you soon and work out what's going on," the beautiful triage nurse said reassuringly before moving away to confer with another nurse.

Suddenly the muttering man that had been behind me stormed up to the triage nurse and yelled loudly. *"This is ridiculous, I am waiting around here visibly needing help and while people like her [pointing at me] who don't even need to be here get spoken to before me!"*

I was speechless and couldn't hold back my tears – thankfully I didn't have to. The nurse stood up from her desk and said sternly, *"You sir, can wait in line like everyone else, you have no clue what that young woman is going through, nor why she is here so don't make assumptions that you are more important! Now you can wait until I call you up!"*

She made a point to come over to the window I was standing at and apologised, *"I am so sorry for his ignorance, trust me we know you're not well."* She smiled warmly, except now I was crying from both gratitude and fear.

It was one of times I wish I looked as sick as I felt. That my 'invisible' cancer could be visible to people.

Soon enough I was taken through and settled into a bed, my nurse took a while to come and see me but it was Christmas after all and I had no doubt they were understaffed. When the nurse trudged in looking unimpressed to be working at Christmas, she just read the file without looking at me. *"So you're having some side-effects to your chemo?"*

I quickly jumped in, *"No it's not chemo actually, I am being treated with new immunotherapy drugs so the side effects are very different."* I handed her the cards that listed all the side effects on them. *"I think I have low cortisol, I've had it once before on my treatment, so if you could do a blood test to check that and my liver function that would be great. There is also a number for my treating hospital if you need any more information."*

She barely looked at the cards I gave her. *"Sure, I'll just need the doctor to write that up which will take a while."*

Mum and I realised it was going to be a long night, I wanted to talk to mum and be alert to know what was going on but I was exhausted. For a busy night, my nurse seemed very disinterested; the nurse's station was right in front of my room, we commented on the fact that she was doing a lot of sitting down in front of a computer and checking her phone instead of attending to her patients and I was a little concerned that I had not seen her contact my team at Peter Mac liked I'd requested.

Almost two hours went by before my bloods were taken, I sighed with relief knowing that those tests would help us all understand what was going on. Finally, with that stress off my shoulders I drifted off with Mum dozing by my side. A few more hours went by and I could see Mum was exhausted so I told her to head home. She wanted to check with the nurse first because if I was going to be moved, scanned or reviewed by doctors in the next few hours then she'd stay. The nurse looked annoyed when she came in and started giving me some results, *"Your blood count is normal, you don't have a fever, I don't really understand why you're in here."*

I was caught by surprise, *"What about my liver function and cortisol levels?"*

She looked at me indignantly, *"They aren't part of the usual set of chemo bloods. But all your results look just fine!"*

"Yes, I would expect that considering I'm not on chemo. So, you haven't tested the two things I asked you to test?" She'd completely overlooked this conversation.

"No I did our usual chemo testing. I can put in a request with the doctor on duty but it's up to him if he clears it." She walked back to her computer and sat down.

I was infuriated knowing once again I was going to have to stomp my feet to be heard here and that might take a while. Mum hugged my tears of frustration away and headed home to sleep while I settled down for the long night.

Thankfully I slept right through until 6am when I heard the nurses doing their hand over. I heard the night nurse say, *"This is Jessica Van*

Zeil, 23 years old, she's experiencing side-effects from chemo."

My insides started to boil! This nurse had spent eight hours with me and still hadn't heard me. I wanted to yell from the top of my lungs for the tenth time, *"I'm not on chemo!"* I was relieved when the new nurse seemed much more receptive as I explained the circumstances to her. The ball started rolling then and by midday on Boxing Day I was on my way to Peter Mac again.

~ Vertigo ~

Emergency rooms are always disconcerting for me, wondering what's happening and why I'm sick; it's a holding place, and for someone desperate to know the answers, that waiting period is tough because it's so stagnant. So I relaxed when I arrived at Peter Mac hospital. I felt at home and was hopeful I'd get some answers and a plan before long. As the day came to a close, I remember watching the most magnificent sunset over Melbourne from my room on the ward. I was so grateful to be there, to have such an incredible view and while the circumstances weren't great, it didn't destroy the beauty or the joy of seeing the sunset. In some ways my circumstances enhanced it, it made the beauty and the gratitude stronger and all encompassing. Maybe it's the contrast of the light and the dark, the joy and the challenges. Without sadness we cannot understand the true beauty and magnitude of joy, we have nothing to make that feeling come alive, to make it beautiful.

As the days passed it felt like Groundhog day, it was the break between Christmas and New Year and the hospital was operating on minimal staff and the whole place was quiet, less patients than I'd ever seen! I had my bloods checked, an MRI done and everything seemed normal yet I was still extremely off balance and dizzy. I escaped to the Youth Cancer Centre as often as I could to get away from the ward.

On my second night my nurse woke me up for my usual check-up; heart rate, blood pressure and a few others. It was three in the morning as I felt the cuff tighten around my arm and release in my sleepy daze, the nurse looked at the results, *"I'm just going to have to check that one again,"* and the cuff tightened and released again.

She kept glancing between me and the machine and I could feel her panicking. *"I'm so sorry, I'm just going to have to check it manually."*

By this point, I was rather awake and curious as to what was going on, the nurse checked it manually twice more before calmly explaining, *"Your blood pressure is really low, I'm sure it's nothing but I am going to have to call a MET call, because if anyone has a systolic blood pressure under 90 we have to. There will be an announcement and shortly after a team of doctors will be in here, I will be here also if you need anything or if you feel overwhelmed, OK?"* I loved the way she handled that, and I felt incredibly calm as I heard the announcement over the speaker.

I was curious, *"When you say low, how low?"*

She smiled at my curiosity. *"81/35, honestly I'm surprised you haven't passed out!"*

My eye widened, *"Wow, I didn't know that was possible, I feel fine, in fact now that I'm awake I might get up for the bathroom."*

She looked a little concerned, *"Careful, you really could pass out!"*

"I'll be fine." I laughed as I stubbornly stumbled into the toilet unassisted. When I stumbled back out I found my room filled with people with clipboards and I was the star of the show. I clambered back to bed and had to undergo another three blood pressure tests just to make sure. I was rather over it by then, I felt fine and just wanted to get back to sleep ... until I locked my eye onto the incredibly hot doctor in the group. Then I was throwing out all the stops, I figured, 'I'm single as all hell, I may as well have a little fun!'

I thought I was being smooth, I asked my very own Dr McDreamy an assortment of questions about the fluid they were using, because it was different to saline and I wanted him to know I was smart, that I got this whole medical thing. In reality, with a blood pressure that low I was delirious as all hell, probably slurring every second word and certainly in no way were my flirtations smooth. I probably looked more like that girl in a club who had had one too many tequila shots and was now flirting with the bouncer! But whatever, it made my night and my MET call a far more exciting experience and one I giggle at every time I think about it!

The doctors believed it was dehydration, which was hard to

swallow (pun not intended!) considering I drink a lot of water every day. However after fluid was pumped into me my blood pressure came back into normal range. The days following were nothing exciting, my bloods came back normal, my MRI/brain looked the same, everything was fine ... which was great except it left everyone a bit stumped as to what was going on!

Finally, I had a neurologist come in to do a bunch of weird tests. I basically fell backwards in bed and had to describe how I felt. I thought it was obvious – even more dizzy. She determined I was experiencing vertigo and that I would need to add another medication to my repertoire. Now the only problem left to solve was why I was suddenly experiencing vertigo; was it a side-effect of the treatment or the surgery? No one wanted to discharge me because we didn't know why, and with the low number of staff and specialists on deck, this could take another week or so!

With New Year's Eve nearing I was desperate to get out. I didn't want to welcome in 2017 while I was in hospital. I'd spent enough time in and out of hospitals in 2016 thank you very much! I think everyone on my team knew that I didn't want to be here, they tried to make it easier by telling me I could see the fireworks and that if we snuck champagne in no one would know but at the end of the day as beautiful as this hospital was, it was still a hospital.

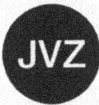

JVZ   **Jessica Van Zeil**   •••
            29 December 2016

Forever trying to escape the ward.
It's been a crazy few days and we are still trying to find the cause of my instability and dizzy spells! I only managed to get an MRI done this morning so fingers crossed for some answers before this evening. In the meantime I will continue to play hide and seek from my nurses in the YouCan centre.
The 29th of December is my youngest sister, Amy's birthday, instead of getting the usual breakfast at home and the birthday girl gets to

dictate the day my family came up to the hospital with all of Amy's presents in tow. I think this was one of the hardest and yet most humbling things for me, to watch everyone's lives get shaken up, to see my family having to make huge concessions for me and to do it without a complaint. I had gotten special clearance to have day leave and go out for lunch to celebrate Amy's birthday, I decided that I could walk the 1km to lunch, except it wasn't 1 km in the end we ended up walking for over half an hour because all the cafes were closed and I was getting tired and extremely hungry! After lunch my siblings walked back to the hospital and I caught a taxi, I was still feeling tired, dizzy and extremely unstable and just wanted to get back into bed while everyone else went to explore the city, I was sad to miss out on the fun but I knew I had to look after myself. While they were out the doctors had a change of heart, they decided to send me home that day, which I was over the moon about!

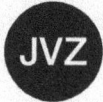

JVZ **Jessica Van Zeil**
29 December 2016 •••

Honey, I'm home.
After an iffy day that was starting to suggest I would be staying in hospital until next week my team of doctors managed to swing things in my favour. We were drawing blanks at every test – thankfully my pituitary gland and hormone levels are fine but cutting those out of the equation made a diagnosis harder.
Turns out I have been experiencing a nasty case of vertigo – while we are still trying to determine the cause this can be done from home with a few more pills to take to keep it under control.

I took it easy once I got home, I knew if I pushed myself and didn't listen I would land myself back in hospital – something I was determined not to do! I was so relieved that all that I had going on was vertigo and while it wasn't nice I could take a medication to help. It wasn't a severe side effect and it wasn't the cancer spreading and that made it a much easier pill to swallow (pun definitely intended). I had managed to avoid all major side effects and to my knowledge I was in the clear for the time being. I celebrated New Year's at home with my Mum and was in bed before midnight. I didn't get to see the New Year in but I was grateful to see 2016 come to a close; at times. I hadn't known if I would and that in itself was milestone!

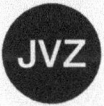

JVZ   **Jessica Van Zeil**   •••
31 December 2016

2016 the year that seems to have turned almost everybody's lives around! I know that all of us are looking forward to seeing this year in the rear view but the last thing I want to do before I say goodbye is thank you.

Thank you for the lessons I've learnt about myself, of my strength, my persistence and my mind. Thank you for showing me how powerfully positive and ridiculously resilient I am. Thank you for showing me the beauty of human nature and humbling me to a point beyond belief. Thank you for making me a better version of myself, teaching me patience, empathy and gratitude – 3 things that seemed like just words that get thrown around but if embraced they can change your entire perspective on life. This year, thanks to so many people we raised enough money to cover my treatment/hospital bills but not only that the fighting we did has helped so many others get the treatment they need and it is now being covered by the PBS!

I have had the pleasure of watching so many people set up their own fundraisers to help me.

Yes this year has been hard but I am grateful for all that it has shown me.

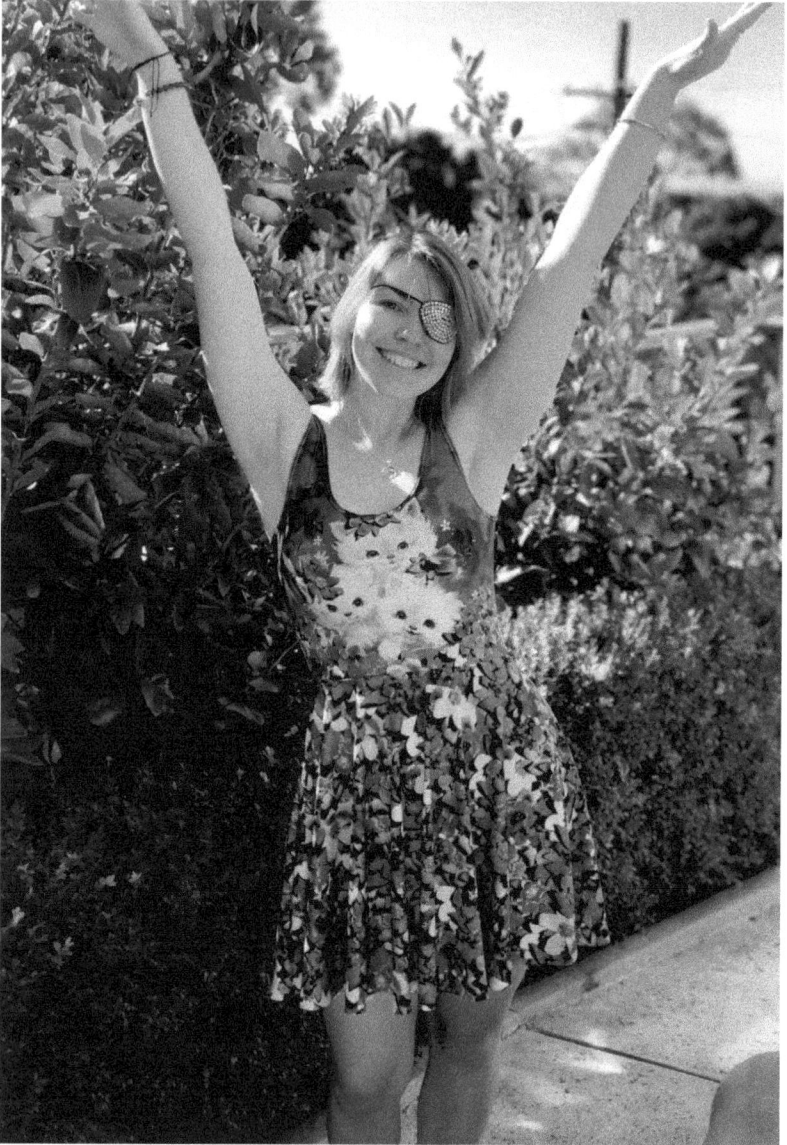

Jess celebrating New Year's Eve.

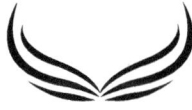

CHAPTER 11

THE HIDDEN BATTLE AND THE PURPLE DRESS

"Persistence and resilience only come from having been given the chance to work through difficult problems."
— *Gever Tulley*

With the start of 2017 I felt brighter and lighter, I was enthusiastic about the future and starting my stabilising treatment. It felt like I had left the worst behind me in last year's basket. It's weird to think that one day can make a year of difference, but that's the power of your mindset. I felt like a weight had lifted and while I wasn't in the clear, I was doing well.

My first dose of single treatment was on the 4th of January. It was a nice surprise how quickly the single dose treatment was, a few hours at most. The risks of side effects associated with this treatment were also a lot lower. I went home with my usual ritual of self-care in mind but straight away I felt a bit off, like something wasn't quite right inside. I didn't have pain, or dizziness but I think part of me just knew. But what could I do? Go to the emergency room and say, *"Hey, can you just watch over me, I don't feel right."* I just had to wait it out and hoped it would pass. So I kept trying to get out, go for a walk or socialise. I spent a great day on my best friend's boat on the 7th of January; we swam, laughed and had fun. While I still didn't feel quite right I put it down to just feeling off after the treatment.

However, the next morning I woke up to a familiar headache and vomiting at 5am. I stumbled to reach the toilet in time, thinking, *"Oh crap!"* Somehow this headache was even more intense than any before. Even after Mum collected all the pain medications we had been given for me to try, I felt no relief! I slipped in and out of consciousness, the only way I found any relief was to keep still and try to sleep. I couldn't look at my phone, or even speak without causing agony. In truth I can't even remember how I got to my local hospital, I just remember the crippling pain, the nausea and the pure fear that this was something far, far worse than any of my previous trips, bar the seizure of course.

I was in a coma-like state and couldn't stay conscious. Mum had to speak on my behalf, explaining my medications, what to test for and also tell everyone to keep their voices down. She was right beside me as they tried painkiller after painkiller and nothing worked. I was in an honest 10/10 pain with tears rolling down my cheek in panic because nothing was working and everything seemed to be taking so long.

Mum stayed with me all day. She didn't want to leave because we had no clue what to expect and she didn't want me to be alone if there was more big news, but good golly, she had to put up with a lot! Every time she moved or ate anything I yelled at her, the crinkle of a chip packet sounded like a blow horn in my ear and only exacerbated the pain!

I remember very little from this time in hospital. The main concern that penetrated my wall of pain was that the doctors wanted me straight on steroids. This however would push back my treatment, so despite the pain, I told them they couldn't start anything without getting clearance from my doctors at Peter Mac along with doing the necessary scans to determine the steroids were actually needed.

I may have sounded calm, cool and assertive but internally I was freaking out at the thought of being on steroids. More specifically the thought of not being on treatment freaked me out beyond explanation! To me, being off treatment meant an increased risk of death, the longer my body had on the treatment the more likely I was to eradicate the disease. I didn't want to be taken off treatment because I wanted to know I had done everything humanly possible to get through this, even if it meant putting up with headaches that were unbearable.

I was in a complete blur; only waking when I had to, only speaking when I needed to. I didn't remember the order of things the way I usually did, the way the rooms looked or even half the things that occurred. When I say I was in a coma-like state, I am not in the slightest bit joking. I was unconscious at least 22 hours of the day, maybe more. Poor mum was terrified, she sat by my bed day in day out for as long as she could because she really did think this might be my end.

At some point during my stay, I was told I had terrible anaemia and that they needed to give me blood. The problem was with my immune system being so reactive it was likely to destroy the blood as soon as it entered my system if it wasn't very closely matched to mine. My brother was there at the time and offered to donate blood on the spot but they said even a sibling can't guarantee a close enough match. They must have found very close matches because I remember having at least two life-saving blood transfusions (thank you to every amazing soul who donates blood because it honestly kept me alive.) Even after the exceptional blood-matching job, the transfusions caused lots of hyper-allergic reactions and hives. My body was still attacking the new blood and my own red blood cell count continued to drop

We were reaching a very dangerous point by then, and after the second transfusion (on my second day in hospital), the doctor put his foot down. He contacted my team at Peter Mac Cancer Centre and repeated that I needed to have the steroids before the side-effects became life-threatening. My other doctors agreed and I knew it was time to move past my fear that the steroids would negatively affect my treatment. I trusted this doctor, and we needed to get this under control straight away.

Forty-eight hours after being admitted, I finally found some relief when a nurse gave me a painkiller they sometimes used during surgery. As the medication hit the pain halved within moments, my face softened and for the first time that day I smiled.

The nurse asked me how I was feeling. I was so desperate to hold onto my new feeling that I remember thinking, 'Be careful what you say here Jess, you don't want her to think you're high – you are high but you don't want her to think that or they might not give you anymore and then you'll be in pain.' So instead I said, *"It's like magic juice, I feel like I'm flying and there's no pain, just nothing, it's amazing and the roof's moving and it's all glittery!"* I rambled on, clearly not giving away at all that the medication had me as high as a kite! It was an immense help and that was the first time my mum heard my voice in days and even better, I was not crying or sleeping!

At another point I had a brain CT followed by an MRI. Thankfully there was no brain bleeds, something I was both extremely surprised and happy to hear. There was however an abnormality around my pituitary gland and the doctors decided to do a lumbar puncture. I was terrified at the thought; can you imagine having someone stick a massive needle into your spine with the aim of drawing out some cerebral spinal fluid? It doesn't sound like a fun time does it? I was much more alert when this happened because of the new medication and probably also the fear. The female doctor performing it had such a calming presence; she talked me through it and before I knew it, it was all over and Dr Calm said everything looked good.

Between the painkillers and the steroids my headache and pain seemed to decrease astronomically, while I was still very uncomfortable I wasn't in agony either and that was a relief. It was also such a great feeling to know what was actually going on, I was having side-effects to my treatment and we had a plan to move forward, which involved more testing, monitoring, painkillers and steroids. Unfortunately there were no beds available at Peter Mac, so I was moved to the oncology ward instead of the emergency department, it was a lot quieter there which was amazing and gave me time to rest, not that I needed it after sleeping for three days straight!

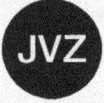

Jessica Van Zeil
11 January 2017

•••

JVZ

Since Saturday I have slept more hours than a koala bear does in a day!

I have been in hospital since Sunday with uncontrollable headaches (not even endone could save me this time) as well as nausea/vomiting and fevers. This little chatterbox couldn't even string a sentence together! We finally got my pain under control late yesterday evening and with a little more investigation we found out that my body was attacking my red blood cells and my liver!

Unfortunately this means that I have to start steroids which may delay my next treatment by a week but at least we caught it early and besides a few very uncomfortable days there are no serious side effects. #notasleepingbeauty

After four days the pain had stabilised, and eventually after running so many tests from bloods, to brain scans, to lumbar punctures, to liver ultrasounds; the oncology team, along with Dr Energiser and my team at the Peter Mac finally had a clear idea of what was going on. I was having side-effects to my treatment, my immune system was heightened and had started to attack my healthy red blood cells as well as the healthy cells in my liver and my pituitary gland. This caused autoimmune hepatitis, meningitis and anaemia.

They decided to send me home with strict instructions to have daily blood tests to ensure that both my liver and my red blood cell count were on the rise with the steroids doing their job. That excited me, to know I could manage this from the comfort of my own home rather than spending time all alone in a hospital being watched like a hawk when in reality it wasn't necessary.

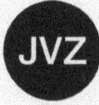

Jessica Van Zeil
12 January 2017

•••

Making it home makes me smile – I swear it's not a side effect of the bag of medications they let me out with.
I'm still struggling with my liver and my blood work but as long as I promise to get blood tests over the weekend and take a long list of drugs and act responsibly, I was allowed out.
Being in the comfort of my own home with my family and my dog brings me the ultimate sense of joy!

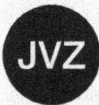

Jessica Van Zeil
18 January 2017

•••

This week's goal of decluttering and reorganising my bedroom complete.
Unfortunately this week has been a little bit crazy for me, from blood tests every day and multiple doctors' appointments we have found that those crazy side effects that were being anticipated had finally occurred! My immune system has been attacking my own body and as a result I have been pulled off treatment and put on steroids to stop any further damage being done – while this sounds like bad news it may in fact be the opposite my body has reacted in the way had hoped and my immune system certainly went into overdrive.
Keeping my mind occupied is very important to me so while the doctors suggested "bed rest" it was more like "make my bed and throw the rest of my crap out!" I'm proud of myself for reorganising everything in my room and sending off about 1/3 of my possessions that I had been shamelessly hoarding for years to the op shop. The result is incredible, a colour palette I love, lots of local art work including @lumak.art@alittlebite_syd as well as my favourite books by @meredithgaston. Now all that's left is a few more finishing touches

on my refurbished wrought iron chair to match the table I refurbished last year.

~ Leave Cancelled ~

Once I got home I kept falling back into old habits of overworking my body and trying to keep the house tidy, in came that controlling cycle again. My obsession got to the point that Mum actually sent me to live with Granny for a while, which was clever because all I had was a book and a clean house, there was nothing I could obsess over and I finally let myself unwind!

A week after being released from hospital, my body was still not fully responding to the steroids, I had turned an odd shade of yellow. I had jaundice as my liver seemed to be getting worse rather than better. I tried to stay calm, hoping and praying that the steroids would dial back my immune system and get my body back on track. On Thursday afternoon, about a week after being at home I got a call from Dr Energiser's team, my nurse angel said that unfortunately the blood tests I were doing daily were not showing signs of my liver function improving, and the reason I was feeling better was because my red blood cell count was on the rise.

My heart sank, helplessness engulfed me. I was trying my best and doing everything I thought was right, eating well, resting, avoiding alcohol, the works. I started searching internally for all the things I must have done wrong for this to not have worked, blaming myself for pushing myself too hard at times, for that glass of champagne I had on New Year's Eve, for trying to keep up with my physio appointments. Of course, all these minor things weren't the reason, in fact it was utter nonsense but at that point I believed it had to be my fault. In some way, it gave me control of my situation, it meant it wasn't random or just a medical anomaly, it put me in charge, even if I didn't know how to fix it. They would keep monitoring me over the next few days, but if they didn't see an improvement, I'd have to be admitted to hospital. Again.

I took that as instructions to be on my best behaviour; resting, napping, relaxing in the hopes of recovering. Much to my dismay on Saturday, Dr Energiser himself called. *"We can't see an improvement, this is getting critical and needs to get under control and the only way I can see that happening is in hospital."*

I agreed, packed my bags full of clothing, books, mindfulness colouring books as well as my laptop, and Mum drove me straight to Peter Mac, where I was immediately put onto a drip with incredibly high doses of steroids.

It was amazing. Within twelve hours I was feeling like me again, full of energy and joy. It's weird, I never realised how sick or exhausted I had become until I felt some level of normality again. It was a glimpse back to what life was actually like when I wasn't feeling snappy, moody, in pain, exhausted and sad. While I never lost my positive streak, it was always a challenge to keep it there especially when I felt the weight of the world ... or even just this disease. It had me crumbling to my knees, it felt like it might be easier to bow my head down, focus on the crap, allow it to take over and infest like it seemed so persistent to try and do.

There was a part of me though that knew I had to keep fighting, that knew no matter how many times I was forced to my knees, I needed to stand back up. No matter how hard it was to keep my head held high I needed to. All because if I didn't, this disease would gain the upper hand, it would be winning, because it would have succeeded at taking out who I really am and would leave me as a shell of myself.

All I had left in this world was who I am, the beautiful, strong, powerful, fun, grateful, joyful Jess. I knew how much I needed to keep being her because I didn't want to see her die out. The words I had heard after I was told the cancer had returned rang through my mind and kept me fighting too.

"It's not your time. Yes, it's going to be a tough journey ahead BUT you still have so much to offer this world. This will not be the end."

And I truly and wholeheartedly believed that I still had a purpose here.

With my love of being outdoors I spent as much time as possible in the hospital's beautiful rooftop gardens taking in the sunshine and fresh air. However this weighed on my mind because I was terrified of the sun and getting burned. I was going through melanoma already and all its horrible and terrifying side effects, the thought of getting to the other side of this and then getting melanoma again was a thing of nightmares! I searched high and low in the hospital for sunscreen and short of buying it there was none readily available.

The quote, 'Be the change you wish to see in the world,' ran through my mind as I decided to put in a letter about this sunscreen issue. In short, I wrote that it was an insult to see 'No Smoking' signs all around the hospital, to have the fact that smoking causes lung cancer thrown in our face at every exit. And yet as patients were encouraged to use the multiple outdoor gardens, it was insensitive that one of the main hospitals treating advanced melanoma, offered no sunscreen in sight! Not to mention, any cancer patient has an increased risk of developing melanoma, so this needed to be amended urgently not only because of the insult in itself, but for the safety factor and the general advocacy to protect your skin, cancer patient or not.

Within three weeks the hospital had sunscreen dispensers everywhere! It was an incredibly proud moment and I respected the hospital for hearing my voice.

The lesson here was to speak up, if you think something is wrong, address it. Most of the time I found it's been an oversight, not done out of spite but your insight can change it. I could have easily just left it as it was and bought my own sunscreen but this way it didn't just help me but also helps hundreds of others who may have thought, 'Oh well, I won't bother saying anything.'

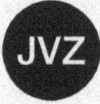

JVZ **Jessica Van Zeil** is at **Peter MacCallum Cancer Centre**
21 January 2017   •••

Hospital bound road trip. I got news this afternoon that my body hasn't taken to the steroids the way we had hoped and while I'm stable there have been no improvements. The doctors plan is to get me back into hospital and get me on some even stronger steroids as quickly as possible.

The last few days I have been feeling helpless, even though I have been doing everything by the book – eat well, lots of water, relax and take every medication prescribed! It's hard knowing that you have done everything in your power and yet your body is not responding (let's be honest the concoction of medications I am currently taking probably aren't helping my emotional state!).

Fingers crossed this little stint in the hospital helps me turn the corner towards recovery. At least I got to enjoy the blue skies the whole drive up to the hospital.

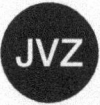

JVZ **Jessica Van Zeil**
22 January 2017   •••

It's safe to say I am feeling much more like myself today! I was so excited to get out into the sun and enjoy the rooftop garden at this beautiful hospital that I am blessed to call my treating hospital.

I was running, skipping and jumping (to the best of my ability) all through the garden as mum just sat and watched laughing at my over enthusiastic attempts at being a ballerina. #canskip

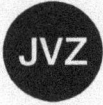

Jessica Van Zeil
24 January 2017

•••

Sometimes we just need to change the way we look at things.
I snapped this quote on Friday when I was feeling a little sorry for myself and the fact I was on "hospital watch" again.

"One way to get the most out of life is to look upon it as an adventure" – William Feather

It shifted my thought pattern from self-pity to a realisation that a trip to the hospital might be what I need to get back to my bright old bubbly self! Sure enough a few days later I'm starting to feel lighter, brighter and more like "Jess" like.
I love flicking through the local author @meredithgaston books filled with beautiful paintings and quotes! They always seem to put everything into perspective and bring a smile to my face.
One thing I have had to realise through my journey is that we can't change the past or even our current situation but we can change our outlook! Take each day as it comes, leave the things we can't change and focus on what is important, live a little bit more in the moment, be accountable for our actions and take pride in the person we are striving to become. Life is such an exciting adventure, and each day we have an opportunity to learn and grow, so why not take it? We were never promised an easy life I can promise you that the journey is worth it.

After four days of extremely high doses of steroids, my liver was still extremely inflamed, so much so the doctors could feel and actually see it protruding under my ribcage, as you can imagine it wasn't too comfortable. Dr Energiser had been in to see me multiple times this stay, which is never a good sign; he was obviously concerned. On the fourth day, he wanted to do a liver biopsy to rule out anything else including a further cancer spread. I was terrified to hear that there was a potential of this, and while he assured me it wasn't likely I had been shown time and time again that my cancer journey didn't seem to follow any of the 'rules' which meant even the impossible might be possible with me.

I had an incredible male nurse who'd been looking after me for days – honestly he had me in fits of laughter the entire time – it was like having a friend on the ward to sass with, who I also knew would wholeheartedly look after me no matter what. He explained the liver biopsy procedure and gave me painkillers beforehand. The team down in the biopsy ward explained that while they could numb the area around the liver, it would feel like a stitch when the needle (which was massive 2-3mm wide!) entered my liver because they cannot control pain in the organ.

They put me on a surgical table, my heart racing, but the team around me made me feel relaxed as they carefully used an ultrasound to locate my liver and the exact spot they wanted the biopsy. Once they were happy they administered the local anaesthetic, and I couldn't feel a thing, phew! They told me to breathe in and brace myself, I was ready for a small amount of stitch-like pain; but it was more like someone had uppercut my liver while holding a jagged piece of glass! I wanted to squirm away but I had to stay perfectly still as they removed the piece of my liver for testing.

Back in my room I felt incredibly sick. The pain was just getting worse and I started running a fever. My amazing nurse was a little worried; he saw the pain painted on my face, my words laced with complaints and discomfort. At one point he remarked, *"I know you don't complain, ever. The fact that you are right now lets me know that you are in an incredible amount of pain and we need to get this sorted!"*

Unfortunately, it took a few hours before he was able to get stronger painkillers. Dr Energiser came up to check in on me and tell me the best news that the biopsy and my liver was cancer free! While I knew the likelihood of the cancer being back was incredibly low, it didn't stop me tearing up with joy and gratitude! He also signed off on my nurse's request for stronger painkillers faster that you can snap your fingers.

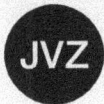

> **JVZ**
>
> **Jessica Van Zeil** is at **Peter MacCallum Cancer Centre**   •••
> 25 January 2017
>
> Stubborn has always been a way to describe my personality and now apparently my liver! My body hasn't been responding to the steroids as quickly as the doctors would have liked so now we are in for a little more investigation.
> I had a liver biopsy done this afternoon and while it wasn't as painful as I expected, it was certainly a very uncomfortable little procedure that I have officially ticked off the bucket list. I could actually feel them going into my liver! Fingers crossed for no more funny procedures and side effects! #cutetummyshots

The next day was Australia Day, a day where usually we would have a family BBQ and relax at home appreciating the beautiful country we live in. My beautiful Mum, Granny and brother came up early with picnic foods in hand to celebrate and make me feel a part of this day. I felt so special and so loved surrounded by my family even though I was stuck in hospital and it wasn't the ideal celebration for them. But they didn't make a fuss and I was grateful for my incredible support network who proved time and time again that nothing was too much for them. I could always lean on them, it didn't matter what was going on, they would move hell and high water to see me smile and make me feel at home and comfortable and involved.

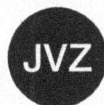

> **JVZ**
>
> **Jessica Van Zeil** is at **Peter MacCallum Cancer Centre**   •••
> 26 January 2017
>
> Proud to be an Aussie.
> Australia Day is a great day to celebrate all that we are blessed with in

this beautiful country! From incredible beaches, supportive networks
and for me an amazing medical system that has made my treatment
and recovery process possible.
Today I would much rather have been celebrating with a cheeky wine
in hand but I know that right now I'm in the right place to get me back
to full health. The wine is on me next year!

A few days later my liver function finally started tracking in the
right direction. This meant I gained a little more freedom over the
upcoming weekend. I had been in a critical state; I don't think the
doctors told me how bad it was until months later; my liver was so
bad it could have failed. I had autoimmune hepatitis, anaemia and
meningitis. Three chronic health conditions with all the crazy side
effects, and if they hadn't responded to the steroids I very well might
not have made it out of that hospital at all.

It was scary to know that my life-saving treatment could have
been the very thing that was my undoing. I don't think I knew how
bad it was at the time, or maybe I did but I didn't focus on it because
I didn't want to feel the stress of it. Hearing that it could have been
the thing that killed me still leaves a horrendous feeling in the pit
of my stomach. The fact is, I have stared death in the face time and
time again and it has changed the way I see the world, the way I
value life. It helps me be compassionate and understanding, but it's
also the driving force for me to constantly be growing and striving
to be the best version of me that I can be. It makes me see every day
as a blessing, it helps me focus on the joy, because even on those days
that were filled with fear and uncertainty I could find joy and I know
there is no reason I can't do that now.

Facing death and coming to terms with mortality is something
that is extremely confronting, it made me realise that all I have
is right now, this moment. While I can wish for years ahead they
weren't guaranteed, that's hard at 23 to realise that maybe all I
had was a day, or a month and honestly, I would be lucky to see out
the year. It took away some of my carefree attitude, because in reality

I wasn't carefree, I was desperate to make the most of every day and I was never ever going to risk my life, I mean really risk it for a bit of short-term fun and enjoyment.

As I sat in hospital contemplating this morality it hit me again how important it was to finish my degree. I wanted to leave a legacy behind if I didn't make it. I wanted to complete something, I wanted to feel like I had done something with my life, that I had actually achieved something, that I had goals I was actively aiming for. That I had an achievement my parents could be proud of. That I stood for something. That I had a vision and future planned out before cancer had come in like a bull in a china shop and tore it all down from the inside out.

When the weekend came I was still in hospital but my doctors finally gave me clearance to have day leave. My younger sister Brittany came to spend some time with me and I was over the moon to get away from the ward. We went out into the city and just went shopping. I was ecstatic to get out and do something normal, and while I was incredibly weak and still had my hospital band on my wrist I felt empowered. As we dotted from shop to shop I got excited walking past a formal dress store with my favourite word plastered out front 'SALE'. We had to go in and have a little look, I immediately realised I wanted a dress to wear for my University Graduation. No, I had not finished my degree but it was going to happen and I was 100%, without a shadow of a doubt going to graduate in June 2017 and I needed the perfect dress to walk across that stage in.

The most fabulous and flamboyant shop assistant welcomed us, a man who knew how to make me feel gorgeous even though I felt rather drab at the time. I picked a few dresses to try on. I looked at myself in the mirror, with my bones protruding, my chest deflated and my face all puffy and round from the steroids, I didn't feel like myself. I didn't feel beautiful. I reminded myself that it was just part of the recovery, about getting better, about moving forward in life. I reminded myself that this incredible body of mine was fighting an unimaginable disease quietly and yet it stayed strong. It was getting better and those medications that were altering my looks were saving my life.

I fell in love with the most incredible red sparkly dress, it was beautiful and I felt like a model as I walked out and saw it glisten over me. I loved a beautiful purple knee length dress too, it sat beautifully and I loved the colour, it was very me. In those dresses and the photos we took I didn't feel like the sick girl from the hospital up the road, I felt like the woman who was going to graduate uni. I asked them to hold the dresses for me and I called Mum. She was a little shocked to hear I had left the hospital let alone the fact that I was trying on dresses for an event that hadn't been confirmed; a goal that she didn't really believe was achievable.

However, she agreed to meet me and take part in my crazy plan that I was concocting. Her answer to the long red dress was a hell no! It was beautiful but it was going to be trouble considering I was still tripping over my feet as I walked, why add another hazard?! When I tried the purple dress on she smiled and fell in love as much as I did. I left with a beautiful dress in hand, its significance wasn't its beauty but what it represented; my massive goal and dream of achieving my degree.

I knew it would sit in my wardrobe for the next six months, that I could look at it in those moments when I questioned my ability to get through this. It was a sign of hope. A reminder that I could achieve whatever I put my mind to, including kicking cancer's butt! That dress still hangs in my wardrobe, and it still holds that meaning. It's a dress with a story; my story. It's a dress with my vision and my goals intertwined in the fabric. It reminds me that I can do anything and everything I dream up, as long as I back up those dreams with action and hard work.

I was discharged from hospital two days later, but before I left I had put the wheels in motion to get my degree finished. I spoke to my study and vocation counsellor at the Youth Cancer Centre and she got to work immediately, speaking to my university and making it happen.

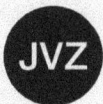

Jessica Van Zeil
30 January 2017

See you later Peter Mac! Thanks for looking after me so well and getting me back home in a timely fashion.

My teddy bear was a present from my family last year when I lost my eye, she is always the part of home I take with me to hospital. Even her jumper was hand knitted by my granny!

Now it's time to rest up and let my body keep recovering! Although I am feeling a million times better I'm still on lots of medications to suppress my immune system and keep me trending to a full recovery.

Caution copious amounts of skipping ahead #happytobehome

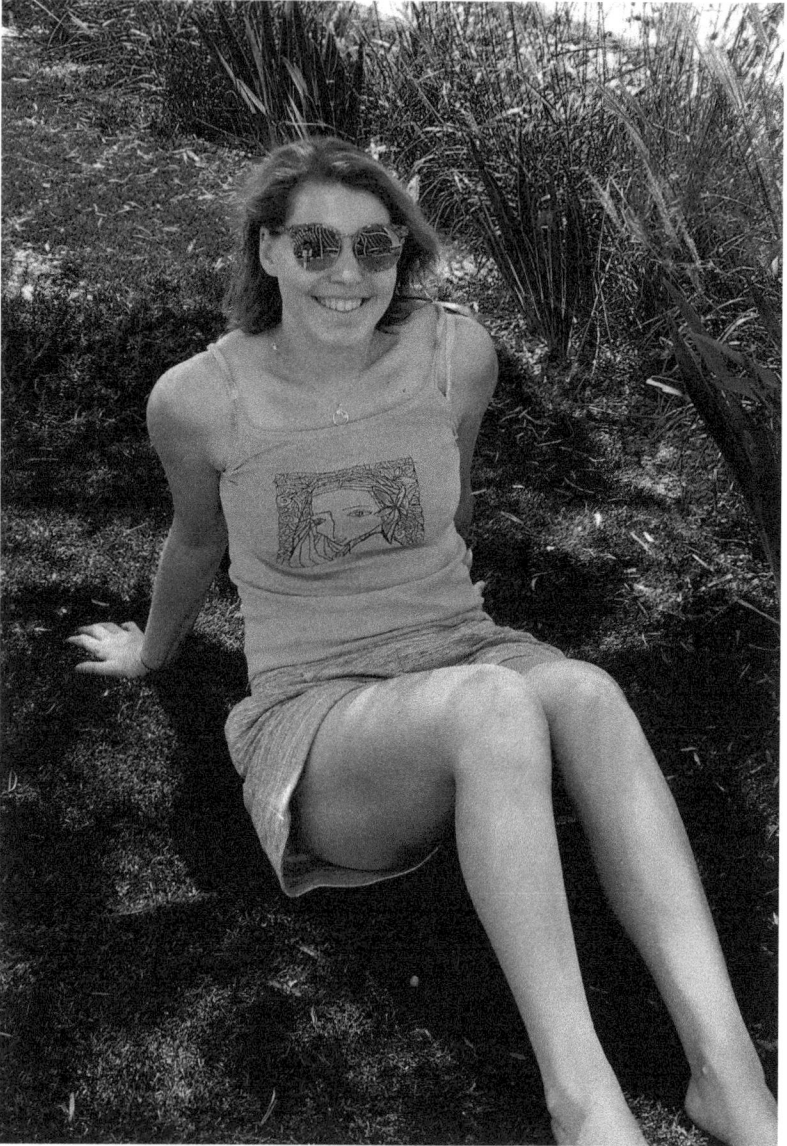

Jess taking a break from skipping around the roof top garden at Peter Mac.

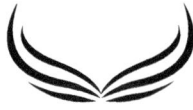

CHAPTER 12

FEAR AND FOCUS

"All we have to decide is what to do with the time that is given us."
— *J.R.R. Tolkien*

The doctors warned me I wasn't out of the woods just yet so when I got home I had to be prepared to take it slow, toning it down to a whole new level. One of the hardest things I came to terms with during this stay in hospital was that maybe I was in over my head hiking the Milford Sound and travelling through New Zealand in a few months. That hit hard. Now, I'm not known for my crying ability I can assure you, but cancer has this cunning way of finding your deepest pleasures and ripping them away without notice. For clawing at your identity and stealing away that things that make you, you.

I cried at the realisation this cancer was going to take away a lot of the things I had loved doing, including travelling. I just didn't feel safe, I didn't know if I would ever feel safe to go away again. It was like a piece of me had been broken, that cancer had deliberately, swiftly and deviously smashed me and the things I loved.

There were so many terrifying variables to confront and deal with, so many 'what ifs', so many medications, so many things that could go wrong, so many things that would put my life at risk. Maybe it was time to accept that life would always be different. I thought that with my treatment ending and my diagnosis being almost five months prior I would be spending less time in hospital and at appointments, but it seemed to be on the rise. I felt cheated.

I got to the point where I couldn't plan ahead, the future was becoming scary and I couldn't guarantee I would be ok or that I wouldn't be admitted back into hospital. Traces of this fear had crept in when I began to feel the effects of the immunotherapy treatment months before. I felt trapped in the vices of this disease again. The side effects had become debilitating and I was missing out on life — *my life*. I hated the idea of disappointing other people if I had to cancel last minute. At least, that's what I told myself.

On a deeper level, it was about protecting myself, managing my own expectations. They were easier to manage when my expectations were low. I was struggling and terrified of the uncertainty of my life. Having low expectations created some certainty and this allowed me to surprise myself and go with the flow. If I was feeling great I could do more and if I wasn't I could dial it back. Expectations are often hard to meet, so trading my expectations of how my day should look for appreciations of what it did look like made it even more beautiful.

I was still exhausted and it took a few weeks for me to regain my strength and for my liver function to restore itself. While I was resting, I fought an inner batter. It was time to start planning life back on my terms but gnawing beneath this hope was the fear that if I planned too far ahead I would end up being disappointed. I was planning a trip to Sydney for a conference in March and was so excited to get out there and do something on my own but I worried how it would go.

I was scared of getting vertigo while flying, I was scared of something happening while I was in another state, all of my confidence and independence that had built up over my life had been stripped back to nothing, back to the beginning like a child's.

It was weird to experience travel anxiety, having every possibility play out in my mind. Just a few years prior I had lived and travelled overseas all on my own. Even though it was hard, I knew how important it was for me to keep pushing my comfort zone and become comfortable with feeling uncomfortable for the sake of personal growth.

My scans in March marked six months since my seizure. The scanxiety I experienced in the lead up was amplified, as if the scanxiety was on steroids, just like I was. Knowing they would determine whether the huge efforts to fight this cancer had worked or whether we'd need a new plan of attack had me totally stressed out. It wasn't so much the 'what ifs' that freaked me out but rather the not knowing.

When the results came back, I posted this message of relief on social media:

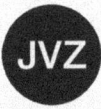

JVZ **Jessica Van Zeil**   •••
6 March 2017

After 6 months filled with surgery, treatment and some insane side effects, my most recent scans have shown no progression of disease! This is a huge relief especially considering how the tumours originally grew so quickly in four months.

Despite this positive sounding post, I want to confess that behind closed doors I honestly hated these results. I did feel relief but I had gone into these scans hoping for a definitive answer, these were built up to be the pinnacle of my treatment and a true indicator of what the future – *my* future – held! When I walked away with no more than a, 'nothing has changed' I felt stuck in a time loop, wondering if things would change, if life would change. If one day I would get more answers or if this was it, if this was all the certainty I could ever expect. Was I going to have to live the rest of my life without being able to plan ahead? The idea tormented me.

While I was grateful to be here at all, this wasn't living, I felt like I was stumbling through life holding my breath. I remember my dad not understanding why I felt so lost, he thought I was being ungrateful, and that hurt; it wasn't like that at all. It wasn't a lack of gratitude; it was just a lack of knowing. It was a hyped-up appointment, one I had put on a pedestal expecting great results or terrible ones. I didn't think at almost six months out we would still be looking at inconclusive results.

If the results were great I could move on with my life, if they were bad it meant it was back to the drawing board. This state of 'no change' gave me nothing, I was falling down a pitch-black hole, not sure if I would keep falling forever or if I was seconds from slamming into the ground.

It meant I couldn't let my guard down; I would always be on edge. Living in fear that every headache could be a spread of the cancer or that I couldn't make plans for months in advance because of that big fat 'what if' hanging over my head. I knew these feelings wouldn't last forever but they stuck around, overwhelming my thoughts and making me feel lost and controlled by this unrelenting disease.

I bravely left for my conference in Sydney, taking the opportunity to visit some of my extended family. This involved a lot of solo travelling on public transport and being completely alone at times with only myself to rely on, both circumstances I had been terrified of only months prior.

After having an amazing trip, I had pushed my body too far and unfortunately, a few days after coming home I ended up back in hospital, which was incredibly disheartening. I wondered if I would ever be able to travel without the backlash of hospitalisation. I didn't want to lose my love of travel, of adventure and being independent.

When I started vomiting and felt the crippling effects of the familiar headaches, I hoped again that this was just another side effect. But already being on steroids made me wonder if this time it was the cancer. I knew there were risks associated with finishing treatment. I was conscious of how quickly my cancer had grown and I had been off treatment for three months, maybe my time was up.

Back in hospital again, I was overwhelmed with both fear and gratitude that if this was my journey starting all over again, at least I had had a chance to enjoy a small window of life and freedom again.

I hated to think what it meant for the future though. I had a trip booked to New Zealand with my mum that was just over two weeks away for her best friend's wedding. I was desperate to see New Zealand, and since I had to cancel Milford Sound, I figured that at least I'd still see New Zealand. I had once again been excitedly anticipating this and now it felt like I was walking a fine line. That belief that maybe I couldn't afford to plan ahead kept sneaking into my mind. So often I had to cancel things when I got sick, I pushed myself too far and it wasn't really worth getting my hopes up to watch them shatter all over again. It was a vicious rollercoaster of emotions and they took their toll on me.

Thankfully after four days I was discharged from hospital, and I nervously packed for my trip with Mum. We were overly cautious this time, considering the turn I took after being in Sydney. We had hospital names, contact numbers, and a bag filled to the brim with medications to help with anything and everything that could happen. I felt safer knowing I was going to be with Mum, if anything went wrong she would be there to hold back my hair or race me to the hospital.

In the end though, we didn't make any panicked dashes to hospital while over there. In fact, this trip was by far one of the best things I have ever done for myself – I was on a high for weeks afterwards! It probably sounds weird considering New Zealand is the closest country I have travelled to but for nearly seven months my life had literally revolved around hospital stays and appointments and not much else. Overseas travel had felt so out of reach and resentment for my situation was creeping in because it had taken away such a huge part of my life.

By finally getting away again, I was taking back some control! I felt strong, empowered and proud of myself for getting back out of my comfort zone and not worrying about the 'what ifs' for a moment and just doing what I wanted to do. I felt so much lighter and brighter to think that I hadn't put my life on hold waiting for when I'm better or more stable. I did come home exhausted and it took a while for my body to recoup but the trip had given me a powerful mental reminder as to what I was fighting for.

~ Live, Survive, Thrive ~

Living with cancer, scanxiety, medication and all the side-effects takes its toll. Hospital visits are relentless and it often feels like a revolving door between hell and gratitude. Hell to go through it and yet grateful to be alive. Even in the calm moments you never feel truly free sometimes, you worry if something is lurking in the background ready to get you.

I found myself in a weird place, I think of it as 'survivorship'. Suddenly I was alone, I no longer needed my doctors and nurses on speed dial, I no longer had people jumping at my every need or desire. My independence had grown so much but the transition felt so sudden that it left me feeling uncomfortable and unsure.

For eight months, I had been wrapped in cotton wool and treated like a porcelain doll and now all that support seemed to have stepped away and I had to come to terms with that and everything I had been through.

My whole life and identity, had been focused on just getting to tomorrow, then next week, then next month. I hadn't had to think about the future, about what I was going to do after all of this was done? When the future suddenly reared up at me I felt so stressed and overwhelmed. I had to come to terms with the fact that I had no guarantee of a future or that the treatment had actually worked. I was being pushed to make plans for the rest of my life when I hadn't even come to terms with the fact that I actually had a life. I hadn't even really dealt with what had happened, I had been in a constant state of fight or flight, I was surviving every day, just reacting to what came up.

When tomorrow isn't guaranteed people swoop in to help, to be there, to support, but as time goes on life keeps moving forward and I felt like I was being left behind. All my friends and family were miles ahead of me and I was just trying to wake up from this reactive slumber I had been living in for so many months.

As soon as I was told I was stable, the people around me expected me to hit the ground running, planning ten years in the future, and having the endurance and capacity to do things. To everyone else my journey was in the past but to me it was a nightmare I was still trying to wake up from. I had felt safe and protected in so many ways and now I felt like a bird being kicked out of its nest and as I plummeted to the ground I didn't know if I could actually open my wings let alone fly.

This was where I had to create my life from the ground up and it was a blessing but also a curse. I was running behind everyone else but also knew deep down that I had learned so much and I needed time to understand these lessons. I freaked out trying to reach everyone else's expectations of me and not knowing what I wanted. Eventually when I sat back I realised I wanted to start living. I had spent most of the last few years in survival mode and I was ready to thrive in life. I didn't know what that looked like or how to go about it but I knew that I wasn't going to live my life on anyone else's terms.

There are long term side-effects I have had to learn to work around and control like spasticity through my right leg that causes the muscles in my leg to over fire and to bounce uncontrollably which makes it hard to walk, run and exercise. As well as a chronic illness called Addison's disease where my body does not produce cortisol, a hormone that is required for normal functionality like waking up, exercising and overcoming infection. Because of this, I have to take a daily dose of steroids which requires me to know my body really well.

These are lingering and difficult, I have no choice but to live with them. I could write a book (yes, another one) simply on the debilitating aftermath of cancer and its myriad of side-effects that are a daily battle — but that's not the book I want to write. Focusing on the hardship only keeps us in survival mode, 'survivorship' but going beyond survival is a whole new ball-game; and one I wanted to play. I just had to invent the rules, or even better, create a new game altogether.

Surviving is just that — survival. It's wonderful and naturally was my only aim. But survival just leaves us there, crawling out from the ashes a bit scarred and bruised, but yes, alive. Survival is about getting by, whereas Thrivorship is about thriving, embracing life and soaring high. 'Survivorship' was lonely and stressful at times but it could also be exciting and invigorating at others. I counted my daily blessings and saw the beauty in how far I had come, and this in turned became my 'Thrivorship'. I used survivorship to protect and nurture myself, to become self-aware and learn the true value of life – my life. But diving into that uncertainty, that unknown state of growth and discomfort every step of the way morphed my life into Thrivorship.

I had spent most of the last few years in survival mode and I was ready to thrive in life. I didn't know what that looked like or how to go about it but I knew that I wasn't going to live my life on anyone else's terms. That wasn't going to be my destiny.

The word 'thrive' originally started around 1200, from a Scandinavian, Old Norse language which translated as "grasp to oneself." And though modern language has also included the terms, flourish and prosper. I love the ancient meaning coupled with our modern-day language. "To grasp to oneself" is necessary. To be there with yourself and hold yourself steady is the ultimate sense of thrivorship. Where you make decisions for your life and stand true.

At first, Thrivorship was challenging and overwhelming, it was personal development to the highest degree because I was in a state of growth and discomfort every step of the way. Discomfort in the sense of being out of my comfort zone. But with time that discomfort became a feeling I craved. I love to continually push myself forward into new unchartered territory without ever losing sight of "grasping to myself", without losing my inner compass or deep inner values and dreams. It meant I was growing, dreaming, thriving. I was truly living!

My life had been burnt to the ground and it was time for the phoenix to rise up from the ashes. I was ready to succeed, ready to make headway into my new life. The phoenix was to rise out of survivorship and into thrivorship.

~ Hats Up in the Air ~

This began with completing one of my major goals. You may recall that at the start of that year, while I was still undergoing my intense treatment, I had set one of my biggest goals; to finish my degree by June! At the time it sounded ludicrous, as I had just spent three of the previous four months in hospital! However, I had made up my mind I was going to graduate, and even went out and bought myself that purple graduation dress that became a visual representation of my goal. I still remember Dr Energiser almost falling off his chair when I told him my plans to finish. While I understood his reaction, my motivation was already set and I wanted to give it my best to get it done! My degree was the only real thing I had committed to in my adult life, and if I were to pass away I wanted to have accomplished it. If I were to survive I didn't want the last semester of university hanging over my head holding me back from living out my dreams.

The amazing Youth Cancer team spoke to the university on my behalf. Explaining my circumstances and my desire to complete my degree as efficiently as possible. My university was amazing, they allowed me to focus on one unit at a time and I only needed to reach 50% of my overall mark before I moved on. This reduced a lot of the time pressure and stress of completing multiple assignments to a deadline; instead I worked to my own set deadlines and aimed to get my assignments in quickly.

Even though the semester and workload were reduced for my situation, this didn't mean it was easy for me. I held very high standards of myself despite the allowances made by the university. I worked so hard and at times ran myself into the ground. In frustration, I often thought about testing my laptop's ability to fly from the balcony, it would 'unfortunately' smash to the ground making me incapable of finishing my assignment. There were so many times I wanted to admit it was too hard and throw in the towel. I remember the tears of frustration at myself for over committing, for pushing myself harder than I should have, for biting off more than I could chew.

In these moments, I would visualise myself walking across the stage in my beautiful dress, embracing the feelings of pride and gratification for accomplishing such a big goal! Finally, after five months, six assessment tasks and nearly losing my mind, I received the message to say I had not only completed my degree in time for the June ceremony but I had been chosen to receive Deakin University's Vice Chancellors Medal of Excellence!

One of my tutors had put my name forward as a candidate, I cried out of pure joy, love, pride, and appreciation. I was completely humbled to know that other people could recognise the hard work and trials I had gone through, not just to complete my degree but to actually be alive.

Graduation day was one of the most surreal experiences of my life; my family and Granny watching proudly from the audience. It was a long day, with practice walks across the stage that was only made harder by my choice (stubborn as always) to wear heels, something I

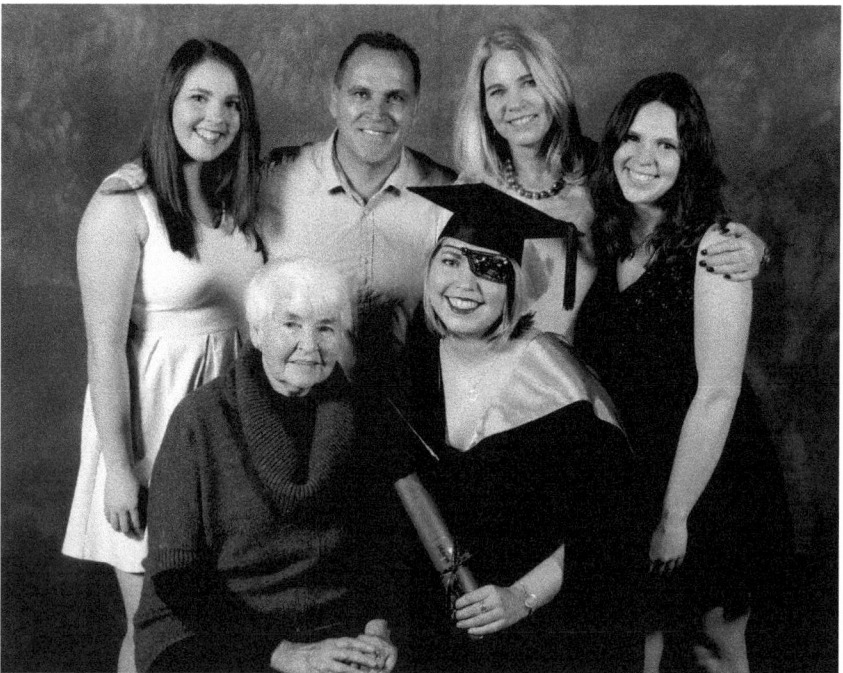

Top (left to right): Amy Van Zeil (sister), Craig Van Zeil (Dad), Heather Van Zeil (Mum), Brittany Van Zeil (sister).
Bottom (left to right): Ann Balshaw (Granny Annie), Jess Van Zeil .

had not done since before my seizure.

When I finally heard my name, I walked to the stage with pride, my head held high. I knew not many people would understand how much this moment meant to me but I knew what it meant. It was a huge accomplishment despite everything I faced. The only moment better than receiving my degree was the second walk across the stage to accept my Medal of Excellence. I was crying; I was exhausted; I felt so incredibly accomplished.

After the excitement of graduation calmed down, I was hit with, 'What's next?' The question made me panic. My career dreams had changed along the way and I knew I didn't want pursue nutrition anymore. I didn't want to get a job, but I also knew I wasn't ready to throw myself into my business. This is actually when I had my biggest melt down. I freaked out because I was not ready for real life. I couldn't fathom the future yet; the end of the year still seemed so far and more like a hopeful desire than a feasible possibility.

I grasped at everything I could. I thought I might study further, perhaps psychology because that would help with my motivational speaking skills for the future. Maybe I could become a psychologist, I was smart enough so why not? In reality, I was trying to avoid dealing with the emotional trauma cancer had caused and having to create a new life, from the ashes around me. I felt lost, uneasy. and all I wanted was security—to have certainty about my future, my whole future. To be able to see what it would look like, to know that I was cured. It wasn't just about not knowing what to do with my life moving forward, it was that I didn't even know where to begin.

Thankfully I took a step back and decided to spend the next few months finding myself, just enjoying and creating my new life. As soon as I made that decision it was like a weight had been lifted. I had given myself permission to just be where I was, to be in that uncertainty and to know it was OK that I was there, that I didn't have to have it all figured out the moment I finished my degree. I spent that time learning to ski, travelling, and I even started dating for the first time in almost two years. Importantly I started investing my time and money into personal development work.

Just being, allowed me such freedom to discover who I was right then, not the Jess I used to be or the Jess I thought I wanted to be but the real me. It was magical to rediscover and create a life from the bottom up. That's the beauty of rock bottom; the only way is up and you can make it look however you want it to.

So, I did return to study but not in the traditional university sense. I studied myself. I learnt about mindset, subjects that interested me and sparked passion. I will forever be grateful that I didn't just jump into another degree because it felt safe, because it was a known outcome. I gave myself time to grow in the direction I chose rather than the direction I thought I should go in. I gave myself time to be me.

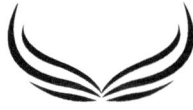

CHAPTER 13

FALLING IN LOVE
WITH ME

*"Owning our story and loving ourselves through that process
is the bravest thing that we'll ever do."*
— Brené Brown

Good golly—the 'L' word.
This journey started even before I was diagnosed with cancer. For a long time, I went looking for my self-worth outside of myself, judging myself through the eyes of a potential Mr Right. But going through the enormity of losing my eye would take pure, inner belief in myself in order to not just survive but thrive. I needed to reflect and focus fully on me, on recovering physically and rebuilding after my emotional breakdown. I needed to learn to love myself, to love the way I looked, to love all that I was going through that would create a new Jess.

In the past, I may have made this sound easy, in reality it was an absolute rollercoaster of emotions. I thought I had a good idea of who I was; fun loving, joyful, grateful, passionate, driven to help people. I wanted to be known for who I was on the inside more than how I looked. A compliment to me was, 'You're smart' or, 'You're funny'; not pretty, sexy or hot. I am a human, a woman and I wanted to be recognised for the value I added to the people around me, not put on a shelf and admired for genetic predisposition or my ability to apply makeup.

All that was easy to say when I was 'normal', when I fitted in with society's standards of beauty. To know I was going through with a surgery that would make me look different, that could potentially cast me out, was an incredible challenge. I literally had to eat my words and prove to myself that I meant what I said. I chose my life over my vanity and I had to live with that choice. I could choose to live in misery, hating the outcome and the way I looked or I could learn to love and appreciate it.

I literally spent 24 hours staring at my bedroom wall contemplating my situation. Eventually, the decision was made. I was going to wear my scars with pride; they were my battle wounds, something to be proud of. I had chosen to live, to be here, I had given up so much for my life and I knew I should be proud of that. I focused my mind on creating positive affirmations, statements that start with, 'I am'. They were claims to my identity, claims to who I want to be known as, *'I am smart. I am beautiful. I am funny. I am confident. I am powerfully positive. I am healthy'.* The list went on and every time I stood in front of the mirror I would say them to myself, affirming those beliefs. To this day, I have my affirmations written on my bathroom mirror in whiteboard marker. I started this before the surgery, to build those inner beliefs before life changed for me.

I didn't want people to pity me; I didn't want them to see me suffering. I wanted them to see me as confident, as owning my situation. I asked myself some important questions around this: 'How do I know someone is confident? What do they look like? How do they carry themselves?'

They stand tall, head held high, they smile, the look at ease, they know they are enough, they are comfortable being who they are and don't care what other people think of them. They smile, they laugh, they exude this positive energy, they command attention, they create eye contact, they believe everything they say and they fully accept who they are.

They walk with energy, like they have a purpose, people want to know them, people want to be them! The reason this was such an important question was because it gave me a reference for what to do on the days I didn't feel confident, the days I felt small and wanted to hide away from the world, the days my head hung low and I avoided looking at anyone. The days when it felt like everyone was staring at me, whispering about me, judging me, because in reality, it was me judging myself. It was my beliefs controlling the situation and this could be positive or negative. It was up to me to decide.

It took a while to get used to my new look, my new style. Having to match in a new fashion accessory to my outfit. Sometimes I loved it, I felt like I was playing dress-ups; other times it felt draining and I wanted to throw in the towel. Again, that was mindset, when I was enjoying it I was focused on the good, the fun, the excitement. When it overwhelmed me, it was because I felt why me; this sucks — it's unfair, I hate this!

The first and most profound lesson I learned in self-love was consciously choosing my words. The words I chose defined the way I would see the world; they defined my reality. The person I had the most conversations with in a day was not my mum, my sister or my best friend; it was me! I needed to own the words I used.

You'll notice through this book the words I use are incredibly expressive, I choose them with purpose, they have a huge impact and it's the way I live my life. I avoid using the word 'hate', it's spiteful and carries a lot of emphasis, yet it's used so freely in today's society. *'I hate banana flavoured ice-cream'* versus, *'Banana flavoured ice-cream wouldn't be my preference'*, similar meanings but one has such heavy, negative connotation that closes down the possibility that maybe there is a banana ice-cream out there that tastes amazing.

I avoid the word 'perfect', because nothing in this world is perfect. It can be amazing, ideal, wonderful but perfect for so many people feels like an unachievable standard and either serves as an excuse not to try or a driving force to continue fixing something that is already excellent.

Even the commonly asked, 'How are you?' Compare the answers, 'I'm fantastic!' versus, 'I'm OK.' The words create our reality.

I found the more I focused on what I liked about myself, gave myself credit for the beauty in me, the more I saw and the more I valued. Even the things I would have classed as my faults or weaknesses became things I saw as either strengths or recognised were things I could focus on to improve. For example, I need to learn to be more patient, however sometimes my impatience means things get done. I can't say I am patient, but I can say I am *practicing* patience.

~ The Best Version of Myself ~

It was just after I lost my eye, at the end of 2015, that I started working with a life coach, Cheryne. In the beginning, I didn't know what coaching was, I looked at it as an alternative to counselling but I really loved it. It was about becoming the best version of myself and building my life back up after cancer had taken out a few buildings. The exciting thing was I could choose how my future looked. I realised my passion was to help people, I didn't know exactly how but at that point it didn't matter. What mattered was I knew what burned in my heart and that was to help and inspire others.

Having a coach was also about having someone to hold me accountable to becoming the best version of myself I could be, it was my own journey, my own life and I got to create it on my terms. I got to experience the value of good coaching and how creating your dream life with determination was a skill that people could learn.

I continued to find more things I loved about myself. I started setting massive goals again. I wanted to work on my health and fitness and started working towards running a half marathon. I could now celebrate my differences rather than hiding behind them. I became so proud of the person I was, I started working on my values, what they were and started living to them. My top value was being powerfully positive which at the time meant being fun, excited, passionate, loving, kind, adventurous, grateful.

I loved the way I look, and I set rules for myself such as no eyepatch at home. Home was my safe place, with family and passing friends that I loved and trusted so I could feel comfortable sharing my new look, my new face with them. I'm not going to say it was easy, I felt naked, like I was baring all but I had to know if they couldn't accept me as I am, a one-eyed wonder, then they weren't really worth my time.

The more time I spent getting comfortable and loving myself the more open I was to sharing photos of me without my eyepatch on social media. I remember the knots in my stomach the first time I posted one. There was elevated fear and worry that people would push back, lash out, be mean. I was scared of being bullied for being different and I was scared this could undo the confidence I had spent so long building. Thankfully the feedback was beautiful, uplifting and positive. I was incredibly surprised but so thankful.

One comment unsettled me. It simply said, 'Eyepatch please.' It didn't actually upset me, but I was alarmed that if this person was saying this to me, imagine who else they were saying things to and how it could affect them. I responded saying *thank you for your input but I love the way I look with and without the eyepatch and will continue to post both.* The strong reactions to the comment from my friends and followers were not as eloquent. A few people told them to get f*&%*d! It was greatly appreciated to see that level of love, loyalty and respect coming from the people I surrounded myself with.

I focused on building my friendships and appreciating the people who had stood by me through everything and celebrating every day. When I was in hospital following my seizure, I gave up the eyepatch all together as it just got in the way and annoyed me rather than making me feel comfortable in myself. I had to face more physical changes with the possibility of being in a wheelchair for the rest of my life, not just looking different but the physical implications of that too. I had to accept that my hair was going to get shaved and a million other things.

The steroids I was prescribed after my brain surgery caused so many side-effects, some hidden and others obvious. My body changed in so many ways, I had gone from looking sickly thin to bloated, moon-faced and uncomfortable as I fluctuated up and down two dress sizes. Not to mention the facial hair, severe acne, and huge increase in allergic reactions. It was through this upheaval that I learned to stop looking at my physical appearance. My insecurities didn't matter at this point, all that mattered was appreciating my beautiful body and all it could do! My body had to relearn to walk and it was doing it! It was recovering beautifully, and fighting the cancer for me. I stopped becoming so attached to the way I looked or the side effects on my body and started just appreciating the fact that my body was working for me!

~ Being Your Own Soul Mate ~

One of the other important lessons I learned was self-care. I had to learn to put myself and my mental health first. My boundaries became extremely strict, there were times when I had to push back quite hard against my parents and friends to keep them in line with my boundaries. If you remember back to those many arguments I had with my dad around not wanting to know statistics, that was one example of many, where I had to execute my boundaries. I didn't want to just be another number or statistic, I wanted to be my own success story and be an inspiration to others who may find themselves in a similar position to myself.

I learned this fancy word, 'No' which I used when I was tired or overwhelmed. I stopped putting pressure on myself to be there and do everything. I finally let go of FOMO (Fear Of Missing Out) realising that if I didn't take care of me and my needs I would have to miss out even more. I learned to accept help from other people whether it was gifts of food or lifts around town. This was incredibly humbling. In reality, I learned to accept myself, as I was, right then. I stopped judging myself. I stopped using the words, 'I should be able to do...' I stopped denying myself the right to be where I was right then, knowing it wasn't permanent.

The foundation was first built during the turmoil of my cancer and recovery. I had spent time learning to love myself, of taking care of myself and making myself my number one priority, I needed to build on it more in order to be the best version of myself. I continued to work on my values and invest in my own personal development. I continued to fall more and more in love with the woman I was, and the woman I was becoming.

Scan times have proven to be the hardest times for me and when I need the most self-love and the most self-care. I find myself unravelling, letting these scans get the better of me. I am so afraid of relapsing, of facing this thing for a third time, and as illogical as it feels and seems, scans are the way I find out if that's happening. As more time goes on, the harder I find scan days and have to deal with 'scanxiety'. With each scan I have created more of my beautiful life and therefore I know there is so much more to lose.

Every week I lay out my goals, I have a planner in place for what I want to achieve. Scan weeks are no different; they just have beautiful, self-care items lathering up my days. The week before I ask myself, 'What do I need?' The list often includes a bath, a massage, mindfulness practice, gym classes, journaling, a walk, a beach visit, cooking something new, seeing friends, reading books. The list could go on and on. This list makes me feel excited and relaxed, it serves to keep me moving forward in my life but focuses in on my health and wellness goals more than business goals.

As I write this chapter, I actually have scans in two days, these will mark two-and-a-half years since my seizure, which is a massive thing but they still terrify me. Just last night I sat in bed crying (ugly crying, 'I can't breathe through the sobs' kind of crying) as I admitted to myself how scared I am. But even within those sobs lies beauty, because as I sob, as I look at why I am scared and it's because my life is incredibly beautiful. I have so much to be grateful for that I am terrified of losing. It's not about dismissing emotions, about banning the emotions I have labelled as 'negative', it's about moving through them, accepting them and understanding where they are coming from. I am sad and scared because I am grateful for everything I have and that's a good thing, I am so blessed to have a life that excites me; one that I fear to lose.

I blogged one of my self-discoveries from that period. I love returning to it and keeping it fresh in my mind.

My Blog

Being single and being happily single are two very different mindsets and I have been both. When I look back at the times where I have been single, I can see a very clear difference from how I used to be and how I am today. The old Jess hated being single, I felt alone, unwanted, uncared for and there was this constant nagging at the back of my mind that kept saying, 'You aren't anyone until somebody else loves you'. It was draining because every date I went on I was looking for the next knight in shining armour to sweep me off my feet and be my perfect match. When they fell short and inevitably ended I was angry, not really at them but that it had happened again. 'What's wrong with me? Why can't I keep a man?' was the mentality I adopted.

It was a vicious cycle that had me either hating men or falling head over heels for a new guy that I had some sort of connection with. It was basic insanity that was driving everything I did, every time I left the house I had to look good because who knows if you will meet Mr. Right shopping for makeup or having coffee with the best friend. I would wake up for uni extra early to make sure I looked perfect for the day or go clubbing and keep my eye out for any potential suitor. BUT for the life of me, I couldn't see the answer staring me blankly in the face: there is nothing wrong with you and there is also no need to hate every man on earth just because it hasn't worked out with a very small handful of them! This is when I realised the elusive 'they' were right when they said, 'to find love you first need to love yourself'!

At the start, I rolled my eyes, how ridiculous and airy fairy is that! Of course, I love myself; hell I treat myself to new shoes regularly! With time however, I have found while I loved my life I hadn't realised that I am not just Jess, I'm amazing! I'm kind, I'm brave, I'm strong, I'm smart and I have a very pretty eye colour ;). The more I focused on my fantastic qualities the more I found. It was like being in a long-term relationship and these findings made me fall deeper and deeper in love with who I am not just the life I live.

This is how I found myself no longer looking for someone else to fill that void and I transformed from being single to happily single. I am now so focused on myself, my goals, my personal development and my life. I am living my life for the most important person, me! I no longer feel dragged down by the constant search for Mr. Right because I have started to live in the moment and started directing all that wasted energy in a new and far more appreciative direction (I love you Channing Tatum but I love me more!).

I know one day I will be blindsided, probably on my left side, by the real Mr. Right but until then I'm going to enjoy being my own soul mate because baby, I'm worth it!

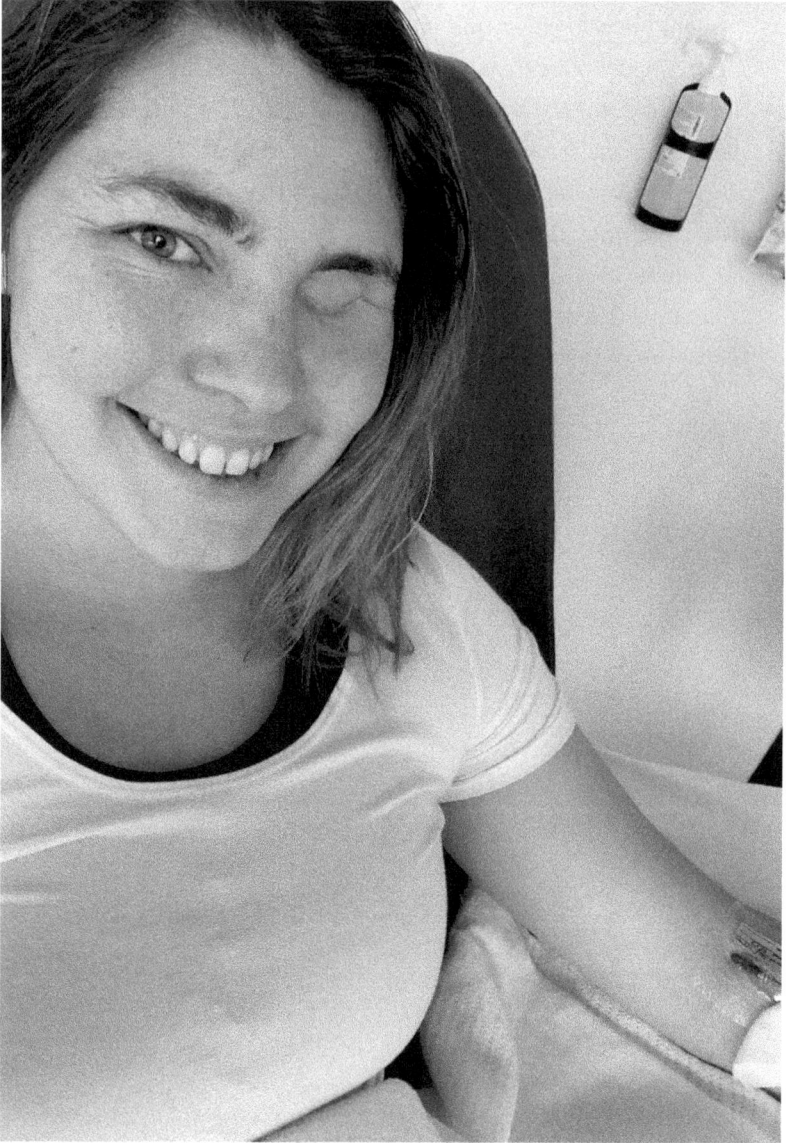

Patiently waiting for scans.

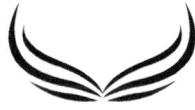

CHAPTER 14

RIDICULOUSLY RESILIENT

"Give me a reason to give up, and I'll give you a reason to keep on. If it's hard and heavy then it's worth something. If it's tired and taxing, then it's moulding you. If you break then it's building you up in a stronger way. So, give me a reason to give up, and I'll tell you why you should not."
— *Madalyn Beck*

Through the peaks and valleys of the last five years, I can't even remember the number of times I was told, 'You're so resilient!' Or how often I was asked how did I manage to bounce back. People seemed to think I had some magical secret hiding in the back of my cupboard but in reality, the only secret I had was that I didn't even really understand what they meant by being resilient. I remember feeling a little baffled, I was just being me, I was just searching for the positives, the way to grow, that was normal – wasn't it?

I felt frustrated because I didn't understand what people were getting at. I even googled, 'What is resilience?'. But all I got was the simple definition, 'the ability to bounce back.' I felt perplexed thinking, 'Well that was self-explanatory!' I wanted the nitty-gritty details, to know exactly what makes one person resilient and another not? How can you tell? What can you do to build a person's resilience? How on earth have I built mine?

I had questions bursting out of me, wanting to know this topic inside and out, because to me it had become second nature. I wanted to be able to help others bounce back from their own challenges and adversity just as fast. I started with a self-analysis; what had I done, what were the steps, what where the traits that helped me build my resilience, helped me bounce back. Then I wanted to know where they came from, how did I build them, they didn't come out of nowhere, (hence the Sundance section of this book). Finally, how can I build them up so in the future I can keep moving forward and embracing challenges in my life.

I found five things I was doing, I then started looking at other people who had faced challenges and adversity, and analysed what they were doing and saying. I threw myself into research and found that the five key traits, skills and tools I had identified were mirrored in their experiences, and backed by research.

As a result, I have created the **PATCH model** for bouncing back, and I'd like to share it with you. PATCH is not just for people with eyepatches, it's a tool for anyone to thrive, whether you're a cancer patient, a teenager, a Mum or even a modern-day pirate (and they don't wear patches by the way). It's a recipe for resilience. A formula that works. How do I know it works? Stay tuned...

~ The PATCH Model ~
Positive. Adventure. Thankful. Create. Honour.

Positive: This is all about mindset. Your mindset is determined by what you choose to give power to! Every single day you will have positive and negative experiences, that's just part of life. Your mind is like a sieve and depending on what you choose to focus on, will determine what is left in the top and what falls away. You can choose to focus on all the crap, the heavy rocks, the things that are going to drag you down both mentally and physically, you can give the power to that one co-worker who said something mean and it can ruin your whole day. Have you noticed that even some of the most blessed people, those rock stars, celebrities who seem to have it all; money, fame, everything they could ever want and yet they are utterly miserable? It's because they have given their power to the rocks in their life, so even though they have countless blessings, they don't count them. What's left in their sieve at the end of the day, the month, the year, are not their blessings, it's their rocks.

When you make a conscious choice to focus on the golden nuggets of the day; the beauty, the joy, the happiness, the blessings you already have, strength will follow. When you give power to these positive moments, you can have the hardest of days, you could even be diagnosed with cancer and yet, you will still find things to be grateful for, the blessings, the lessons, the growth opportunities.

That doesn't mean you won't experience sadness, anger, anxiety or stress, they are emotions that you will face and need to address, but focusing on those golden nuggets helps you move through those emotions quickly and live in a state of joy and gratitude.

> 'When you change the way you look at things, the things you look at change.'
> — Dr Wayne Dyer

By changing your mindset, your focus will change the way you remember things, it will change the way you view your life. I see my experience with cancer as a challenging but beautiful experience. Not something I would ever wish on anyone else but also not something I would take back. I remember the kindness of my medical team, the laughter I shared with nurses, the joy I felt when I lifted my leg off the bed for the first time, the humbling feeling of support from all the people who donated to my treatment, the beauty in the sunsets I saw from my hospital bed. It doesn't diminish the challenges I had but the meaning I have created out of my experience is something positive, I have given life to the beauty and moved through the challenges and as a result that's what I hold onto.

Adventure: Life is an adventure, filled with learning, challenges, beauty, ups and downs, love and pain. However, you get to choose whether you embrace that adventure, those challenges, sometimes even seek them out, or stay inside your comfort zone where it's safe, only getting pushed out of it when you absolutely have no other choice and even then, you're going to grumble the whole damn way.

Is your focus on the patch of grass at your feet? Is your head down? Are you wanting to stay safe within your beliefs, within your little bubble? Is your life based on staying safely within familiar boundaries? When challenges happen, they ask *why me?* They focus on all the things they are missing out on, why they can't do or achieve. The questions they ask themselves aren't there to build them up and find solutions but more to validate their preconceived ideas and opinions of the world that are very ridged. They have a closed mindset.

Alternatively, is your head up curiously searching for new opportunities? Asking empowering questions that help you grow, change and develop as a person? They aren't discouraged by failure but look at it as an opportunity to grow and learn so that next time they try they can improve. They are not easily disheartened, they are adventurous, seeking out challenges and thriving on growth and moving forward. They are resourceful and have a, 'never give up' attitude. The questions they ask themselves are, 'How else could I do this? What else could this mean?' They have a growth mindset.

> *'It's not a lack of resources but a lack of resourcefulness that stops us.'*
> — *Tony Robbins*

Thankful: Being thankful and practicing gratitude is something that changed my life. In today's day and age, media and marketing train us to constantly want, and believe that in order to be happy we need the latest phone/iPad/dress (insert whatever you think you *need* right now). It takes our focus away from what we already have —the people, the random acts of kindness, the love, the memories, the treasures because we are focused on the next superficial thing.

Practicing gratitude brings us into the present, it allows us to refocus on what has meaning and gives us an opportunity to truly appreciate the people and the things we have in our lives. Daily gratitude practice has been shown to improve our health and wellness, our relationships, our performance and increase a person's happiness by 10% (that's the same increase as doubling your income!). I used gratitude every day while I was in hospital, and every day since. I have changed the practices I use to do it, from journaling, to gratitude jars and sharing my three gratitudes with another person or people.

I started journaling to make my granny happy. She gifted all her grandkids with one many years ago and although I thought it was silly and pointless I wanted to make my granny smile. I started with one thing and the lists eventually got so long I had to put a cap of my three things I was MOST grateful for. Since 2014 I have created my own gratitude journal and have it as a special bonus in the downloadable content.

Gratitude jars are fun and something I have recently gotten into. Every day for a year you add something to your gratitude jar, you can challenge a whole group to do it, whether it's your whole household or a group of friends and once a year, or even a few times a year you come together for 'thanksgiving' dinner and each share your jars. Alternatively, you can do this on your own, fill the jar up with one gratitude each day, more if you'd like, and on days when you are feeling down, stressed out or anxious, you can open up the jar to remind yourself of all the beauty in your life.

Sharing three gratitudes over dinner or before bed with a loved one is my favourite. It's a beautiful insight into each other's lives and what we are appreciating throughout the day, about each other and about other people. It gives us a platform to appreciate life and our experiences, sometimes we have similar things we are grateful for and other days they are so different it's insane!

I also share my gratitude on social media with the #iamgratefulfor so join in on the fun, I'd love to see what you're grateful for!

My favourite thing about practicing gratitude is that the more often you do it, the more you will find in your life to be grateful for. At the start it might feel like an uphill battle but with time it will snowball and you can choose to live in a state of gratitude.

Create: Creating the life of your dreams requires a vision and a blueprint, to do that you need to set goals, so that you have a target to aim for. So, the first thing I always get asked is, 'What areas of my life should I set goals in?' The answer is simply any area you value or that's important to you. If you aren't giving energy and focus to something that's important, your resources – being your time, your money and your energy – will go into something less valuable and lasting.

What's the difference between goals and dreams? Goals are just dreams that have been backed by accountability and action. Accountability focuses on two areas; first being to set a deadline that you are aiming to achieve your goal by. The second is to shout it from the rooftops, tell everyone. Tell your coach, tell your friends, tell your family, heck, even tell your neighbour's dog. That way, when you don't feel like doing it or you get off track, you have someone to hold you accountable and pull your focus back. OK, maybe the dog won't hold you accountable — but tell him anyway.

Back your goals by action! Firstly, it's about making them measurable, if your goal is to make more money, is that $5 or $5000? Because that's a big difference and you need to be specific! Is that per week, per month, per year or over your lifetime? If your goal is to be happier, ask yourself, 'happier compared to what?' If you were to rate your happiness out of 10 right now, what's your answer, and what do you want it to be. E.g. I feel 5/10 on my happiness scale right now and I want to be an 8/10. I will know I have reached that when I laugh ten times a day, when I smile a lot more, when I have built a positive mindset and I am doing gratitude journals every day.

Then it's about deciding your actions, what do you need to do in order to move towards your goal.

The last part of this is grit, the ability and willingness to stick to a goal even when the excitement wears off and challenges or road blocks arise. The best way I have found to cultivate grit is by having a strong WHY. The driving force and reason I absolutely must achieve this goal and nothing will get in my way. It's the reason you practice, you push yourself, you keep putting in the hard yards.

Setting big goals is half the fun, you want them to scare you a little, maybe even make you wonder if it's possible. Then it's about breaking it down, how will I know I am on track?

Invest in your goals and your dreams, when I set a massive goal I always ensure I have the right coach supporting me on my journey, someone I can trust to keep me on track and push me to achieve my goals. I have seen what I thought were five-year goals for myself come together in six months!

Setting goals and working towards them makes me feel so fulfilled and uplifted, it builds my confidence, my self-belief and makes me strive to be a better version of myself. Remember also, it's not always about reaching the goal, the fun part, the real beauty is about the growth we go through along the way. Fear is temporary, regret lasts forever: don't let your fears hold you back from creating the life of your dreams.

Download my **FREE Goal-setting Workbook** at
deanpublishing/eyewon

Honour: This is all about honouring yourself. It's about self-love, building yourself up, being conscious of the words you use, the way you describe yourself. You must always be in your own corner, be your own cheerleader, build yourself up. It starts small, creating positive affirmations; using those, 'I am' statements and owning them. Then comes setting your values, asking who am I and what do I stand for? What do I want to be remembered as, and ensuring that your actions reflect them, don't tell yourself you're honest and then lie to someone's face. Finally make sure your investment of your resources; time, money and energy also reflect your values. If family is your number one value then don't spend all your time working.

Believe in yourself. Be your own cheerleader. Know that you are completely capable of achieving what you set your mind to and never give up. Embrace that, 'never give up' attitude and tune out the noise of self-doubt and other people's doubts. Know that when someone says, 'That's impossible', it's not about their lack of belief in you but rather the lack of belief in themselves. They would never push themselves to that extent so they can't imagine anyone else being able to do so. Whenever I hear someone say, 'You can't do that', 'You're crazy', or 'That's impossible.' I simply smile and use it to fuel my fire, I take it as a challenge to not only prove them wrong but to also inspire them, to show them and myself that anything is possible.

> *'What other people think of you is none of your business'*
> — *Deepak Chopra*

Self-care is about filling your own cup and knowing that it's not selfish but rather necessary because you cannot pour from an empty cup. Do something for yourself every day that makes you feel happy, appreciated and loved. Whether it's an hour-long bath or a ten-minute walk around the block. Ask yourself what do I need?

I have found great value in creating my own personalised "self-care toolbox". I have a list of all the things that calm me down and bring me joy. I have it sectioned off into short, moderate and long tasks and I have about ten items under each. When I am feeling in need of some self-care, I can look over the list and choose. I have also shared this list with some of my loved ones so they can help me out if they notice I am feeling a bit empty and need something to fill me up.

Set boundaries, protect your energy, your time, your money, don't feel like you should be seeing this person or should be buying that raffle ticket, if it's not important to you, if it's not of value, if it's not serving you or in alignment of your values, then don't let it take your special resources! Don't be afraid to say no. For two small letters, it can be a powerful word.

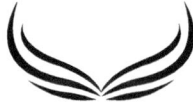

CHAPTER 15

MY SUNDANCE

"Turn your wounds into wisdom."
— *Oprah Winfrey*

One of the statements I hear often is "you must have always been that resilient!" While it sounds flattering it implies two things. The first is that I was born with some 'resilient gene' or have some special talent for overcoming adversity. The truth is I have neither. In reality what I have is actively implemented many daily practices and resilience tools and skills into my life.

The second assumption is, 'I wouldn't be able to do that!' And that's just not true, you would. You can learn to cultivate resilience. That's the method that works. Don't wait to be resilient spontaneously — it won't drop down from the skies and land in your mind like a beaming miracle. You need to believe that you can overcome every challenge you face, that's why building your resilience and pushing yourself outside of your comfort zone is so incredibly important!

I like to think of life like a Sundance. An incredible, intense experience filled with agony and ecstasy, ups and downs, life and death. A Sundance is part of the indigenous people of the USA's rich history, where a chosen group put themselves through unimaginable circumstances like fasting for days on end as they dance around embracing whatever conditions Mother Nature throws their way as well as piercings. It is seen as both a sacrifice and a learning experience, one that they learn perspective and tools to take into the future.

We don't have to be Native American to see life as a Sundance. To see that the harsh experiences make up our life too and that beautiful blessings can arise from insurmountable circumstances.

An indigenous elder once said, "Sometimes we don't see it right away but we know that as we go through life and we look back, all those things that we've gone through give you the strength but the ceremonies make you proud of who you are."

Yes, the ceremonies, the initiations, the good and bad times all shape us. Our accomplishments and our so-called failures – make us who we are today.

He said, "what we're passing on to the youth, we're showing them that there is an end to the means of what they are going through, and whatever they are going through at that particular time it's a learning and once you get past that point it gives them strength. It's taking the good and the bad and that's what makes your path in life."

My Sundance, my experience of hell and heaven showed me what I was capable of. What we are all capable of. That the past and all those experiences shaped me, and yours shape you too.

"To watch us dance is to hear our hearts speak"
— *Derrick "Suwaima" Davis, Hopi/Chocktaw*

My Sundance was precisely that. It revealed my heart and allowed it to speak in a way that words couldn't.

When I take time to reflect on all the experiences that happened in my life, I can now see them differently. I can see them as part of my Sundance. Part of my initiation into being the powerfully positive and ridiculously resilient woman I am today.

Here is my Sundance. All the parts of me, my life and my experiences that I no longer see as 'good' or 'bad' as 'positive' or 'negative' – because they now all swim in the delight on one dance – mine. Yes, I am Jess Van Zeil and this is my Sundance. (Cue some

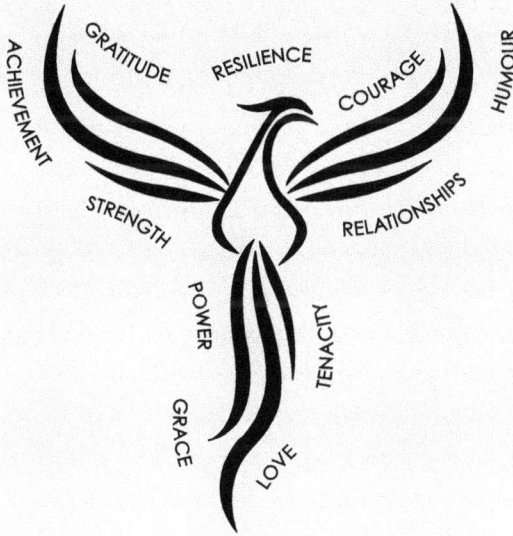

GRATITUDE RESILIENCE COURAGE HUMOUR ACHIEVEMENT STRENGTH RELATIONSHIPS POWER TENACITY GRACE LOVE

Every time I danced around the fire, I got burned, but like a Phoenix I rose from the ashes, each time getting stronger than the last.
I used all these life experiences in the fire as building blocks to get my wings. They are all part of my unique Sundance.

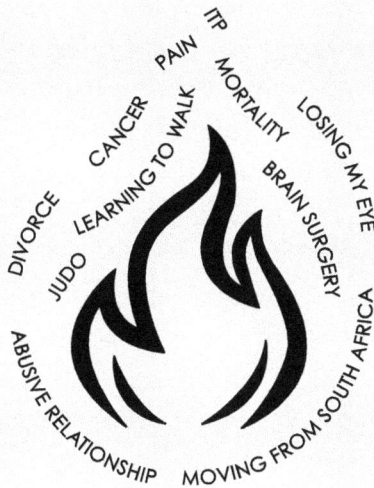

ITP PAIN MORTALITY CANCER LOSING MY EYE DIVORCE LEARNING TO WALK BRAIN SURGERY JUDO ABUSIVE RELATIONSHIP MOVING FROM SOUTH AFRICA

inspirational music here as we begin to create your Sundance too).

Reflecting on my Sundance in my early life, I was surrounded by the unconditional love of my parents who were always close-by. But I also remember being different — having bruises on my body, having to wear a helmet and regular trips to the hospital, I didn't understand why and remember craving to fit in.

My mother, Heather, went to hell and back trying to protect me. This is her story, part of her Sundance (and mine), in her own voice.

~ Jess: My Miracle ~

Jess has always been a fighter and a survivor. Before she was even born she was fighting the odds of survival. After five long years of trying to conceive, I finally fell pregnant through IVF. I was absolutely overjoyed I was finally going to have a baby! I couldn't contain myself and told everyone my wonderful news.

My initial joy quickly turned to dismay when at nine weeks I started spotting. I was absolutely convinced I was going to lose this precious child I was carrying. I rushed to the doctors for a scan and was relieved to see and hear her tiny heartbeat. I was booked off work and told to take things easy, by eleven weeks the spotting had stopped and I started to think my problems were over; I had reached that magical twelve-week mark.

That same week I suffered a massive bleed, I was devastated, sure that it was all over this time. It was back to the doctors for another scan which I thought would just confirm my worst fears, but there was tiny tenacious Jess alive and kicking away totally unaware of all the stress she had caused! I did however have to spend the next three months confined to bed as this was now deemed a high-risk pregnancy.

When Jess finally arrived on the 7th of July 1993, this too wasn't without a bit of drama. After a long exhausting labour Jess appeared to be going into stress so the decision was made to deliver her by C-section. Everyone was getting prepped and ready, when Madam Jess decided she would rather come naturally! Not a good idea – the umbilical cord was wrapped around her neck twice, which meant she was literally being strangled as I tried to push her out. I knew things weren't going to plan and it seemed like ages before Jess let out her first wail – I have never been as pleased as I was then to hear a baby cry! If it hadn't been for the quick intervention of my gynaecologist we could easily have lost her at that point.

At 18 months old, Jess had a very close brush with death; she fell into our pool unnoticed and almost drowned. Jess had had a lovely afternoon swimming with her dad. When they were finished, Craig took her out and dried her off; then he turned back into the pool to reattach the pool cleaner. Jess must have followed him, and silently launched herself off the step in an attempt to reach him, but without her armbands on, she just sank. When Craig turned around to get out he noticed Jess had disappeared, he was just about to go looking for her when he noticed her lying motionless on the bottom of the pool. I can only imagine what went through his head in the split second before he pulled her out; she was already blue! Mercifully he managed to revive her. The rest of that day we both anxiously watched over her, replaying over and over what could have been the worst day of our lives.

A couple of months after Jess turned two, on a Friday afternoon I noticed a bright red rash all over her chest and neck. I panicked because earlier that day I had noticed a nasty bite on her face, and now presumed she had been bitten by a spider and was having some kind of an allergic reaction. I immediately called the doctors rooms and when I described her symptoms they insisted I bring her straight in. On examining her, the doctor asked if I had noticed any unusual bruising. Remembering an incident from the day before I showed him a very nasty raised bruise on Jess's arm. He asked how it had happened and I explained that she had been in the care of her nanny. When I had questioned her, she said she had no idea how it had happened. I had been very upset, as in my opinion there was no way anyone could get a bruise like that without knowing how it had happened!

The doctor then told me he suspected Jess might have something called ITP, which at that point meant nothing to me. He didn't go into too much detail, as he first wanted to confirm his diagnosis with a blood test, although he did say that if I was at all worried about Jess over the weekend to call him immediately. We were then sent down to pathology for blood tests, and told to call the surgery on Monday for the results.

We didn't have the internet back then, so at that point I was totally oblivious to the seriousness of Jess's condition. But by Sunday morning, I knew something was wrong, Jess was covered in bruises, and in places you don't usually get bruises! That afternoon we had to attend the christening of a very close friend's first child. It was a very warm day and Jess ended up going for a swim. With her bruised bare skin exposed she soon became the focus of all sorts of questions, most of which I couldn't answer. I was later horrified to learn that one of the guests had suggested to my friend that Jess might be a victim of abuse and that perhaps she should call child services (I soon learnt this was a very common misconception).

On the Monday before I could call the doctor, I received an urgent call from the surgery asking me to bring Jess straight in. I wasn't sure what to expect but I knew it wasn't good. I remember sitting anxiously in the doctor's room with Jess on my lap, being told her platelet count was 26 (normal being 150-450), that the rash was not a rash, but actually burst blood vessels under her skin. Whilst listening and trying to take in all the doctor was saying, Jess's nose started to bleed, I didn't know at the time but this was another sign of her condition.

The rest of the day was a blur; I had to take Jess down to pathology for more blood tests. Friday had been bad enough when Jess didn't know what to expect, but on Monday as soon as Jess realised where we were going she ran off screaming, 'No, no, no!' I felt like a monster holding my hysterical baby down while they drew blood. By the time it was finally over, I was shaking and very close to tears myself. An emergency appointment had been set up with a paediatric haematologist, whom we saw as soon as the results from the blood tests were available. Jess's platelet count had dropped even lower and was now only 6! I felt so out of control and helpless; being told your child has a life-threatening condition, that a blow to her head could cause a potentially fatal cerebral bleed! I just felt numb, I was being told Jess needed to have a bone marrow biopsy, to rule out haemophilia and to ensure her bone marrow was functioning normally, and that they wanted to do it that evening!

Up until that point it had just been Jess and I, but with this news, I called my husband with a list of things he needed to bring to the hospital. I was so thankful when he finally arrived; a burden shared really is a burden halved! Later that evening it was confirmed Jess had ITP (Idiopathic Thrombocytopenic Purpura), a blood disorder where your immune system destroys its own platelets. She was immediately started on a course of corticosteroids – which reduces the activity of the immune system.

The six weeks that followed were extremely stressful, trying to contain a very active two-year-old, when you have been told a knock to her head could cause a cerebral bleed, was exhausting. Just as challenging was actually getting Jess to take the cortisone, it was in a liquid form and was the most bitter thing I have ever tasted. I soon realized there was no way Jess was going to take her medicine voluntarily. After several failed attempts, I finally found the only thing that worked was to add copious amounts of strawberry Nesquik to a 250ml bottle of milk (this was the only flavour that seemed to disguise the taste of the cortisone).

Besides the challenge of getting her to take her medicine and the stress of constantly watching over her, the physical effects of the cortisone on Jess weren't pleasant either. Everybody talks about the Terrible Two's but this was literally your worst nightmare – a two-year-old on steroids! Before I had always been able to reason with Jess, but on steroids this became impossible. She was always irritable and grumpy, she was that child that screamed when she didn't get what she wanted at the supermarket, the one who wouldn't share, who answered, 'No!' to every question. Her behaviour was met with lots of eye rolling everywhere we went; thank goodness it wasn't permanent!

In most cases once you are weaned off the cortisone your immune system reverts to normal, but unfortunately in 5% of all cases there are more long-term effects, and Jess was in that 5%! After completing the six-week course we returned to the haematologist, which also involved another visit to pathology. This went a bit better than our previous visit – I was learning the subtle art of bribery, and there was a very conveniently placed vending machine right outside the pathologists. Jess's platelet count had risen, but was still only 35 and the tell-tale bruising was still very evident. Her specialist Dr Con explained to us, that as she had not responded sufficiently to the initial treatment they would have to continue to monitor her very closely.

The reality being she had a life-threatening condition, and until her platelet count was back to normal, we would have to go for weekly check-ups at the paediatric oncology and haematology unit at the Johannnesburg General Hospital. I don't think I ever fully accepted that what Jess had, was potentially fatal. Most of the kids at the unit looked much sicker than Jess and when I was told she was eligible to sign up for the Make a Wish Foundation (a group that grants wishes to terminally ill children) I refused.

We soon got into a weekly routine, our first stop was the nurse who took the blood samples (thankfully this was not as traumatic as our previous experiences had been). There was a wonderful nurse called Julia, all the children loved her, she always had the biggest smile and had the most amazing way with children, she seemed to know all their names. Each child had to have their finger pricked, and a small sample of blood drawn, and the only time there were ever any tears, was when nurse Julia wasn't there! She made them choose which finger was going to be pricked, and after receiving the mandatory Band-Aid and a stamp, it was up to the clinic to wait for the results before seeing the doctor.

Not a particularly fun place to visit, but Jess loved it! There was a wonderful array of toys, and a group of volunteers who came every morning and ran activities for the kids. Friday was baking, which Jess loved so we got into the habit of going to clinic on Fridays (I think this is what instilled a passion for food and cooking in Jess, which she still has today). These visits were mostly uneventful and the only time they intervened was when Jess's count got below 20.

I am not sure why but they seemed to alternate treatment methods, so when Jess's count dropped to 18 a couple of weeks after her initial treatment, she was given a mix of platelets intravenously.

As the treatment was done over three days they inserted a cannula and left it in, I was initially grateful for this as I thought it meant she would only have to endure being pricked once. But after the second day's treatment, I noticed the bandage around her hand was was soaked in blood and I had to rush her back to hospital. I was terrified they wouldn't be able to stop the bleeding but Jess didn't seem at all concerned.

Unfortunately, the cannula had to be removed and a new one inserted the following day, I wasn't allowed in when they did it but I certainly heard Jess screaming. Over the next two years Jess got used to being pricked and I remember sitting next to her the last time she had to have a cannula inserted, she was almost four and she just sat and watched as they pushed it in and didn't even flinch!

When Jess was three I had asked the doctor if it would be possible for her to attend preschool as all her friends had already started. I was given the go ahead, but soon found out it wasn't going to be easy; none of the schools I approached were prepared to take her on. I did however eventually find a small Montessori playgroup with the most amazing owner Laurie who agreed to take Jess. Laurie was nervous, but a close friend of hers had a haemophiliac son whom had never been able to attend preschool, and Laurie knew if she didn't take Jess no one would.

Jess loved playgroup even though she had to wear a bike helmet whenever she played outside, and wasn't allowed to play on any equipment over a meter high, a cerebral bleed was still a very real danger. Jess never fussed about wearing her helmet, a couple of the other kids even wanted to wear them too. However, to Laurie's dismay, she was the most daring and adventurous kid in the school, which thankfully only ever resulted in some very nasty bruises. I don't have any pictures of Jess wearing her helmet; I think I was more self-conscious of her standing out than she was.

The helmet wasn't the only thing that highlighted Jess's condition; she was also always covered in bruises. People used to stare, and would often ask Jess how she got so many bruises. I often felt judged, as I am sure many people suspected she might be abused. Jess had an exceptional vocabulary for a small child, so I told her if anyone asked, to tell them she had ITP, which made her bruise very easily. This seemed to work, as the critical stares turned to sympathy.

During this time, although I was constantly aware of Jess's condition, life went on. We travelled overseas with her to attend my sister's wedding, which involved more than the usual planning, as we had to factor in Jess's weekly blood tests. We managed to organise a mobile nurse to come to the place where we were staying, but unfortunately, they needed to take a proper blood sample every time, so I again stooped to bribery to try and get Jess to cooperate. Staying with family made things a lot easier as I had a lot of support and despite everything had a wonderful trip.

Soon after this trip, and another bout of IVF I fell pregnant with twins. Our weekly visits to the hospital continued and as I neared the end of my pregnancy I found these visits rather taxing, on one particular visit (possibly the last before the twins were born) we had gone in for our routine visit only to be told Jess's count was 19 and she required a transfusion of platelets. I hadn't been prepared to spend the day and was absolutely exhausted by the time we left eight hours later. Jess must have been too, but as the unit was so well equipped with books and toys she never seemed to mind spending time there.

After the babies were born Jess enjoyed our weekly visits to the hospital even more, as she had me to herself! I tried not to molly coddle Jess, but the underlying fear of her condition often used to kick in and I would find myself jumping up to protect her. I think this irritated Jess and made her fiercely independent, as I recall her telling me on more than one occasion, 'Leave me alone, I can do it on my own!'

When Jess was almost four I had a conversation with her specialist, I wanted to know if Jess's condition could be permanent. I was told at this point that it was possible (but very rare) and the only treatment they had found that worked was removing the spleen, but that they would not consider doing this until she was 10 – not very encouraging news. But fortunately, not long after that Jess's count started going up and about a month after her 4th birthday, we were given the wonderful news that Jess's count was 145 and we didn't have to go to the clinic weekly anymore! We had one more follow up with the specialist six-weeks later and Jess was given the all clear – you cannot believe the relief I felt that it was over!

At the age of 10 Jess cheated death again – we were at the airport and her dad asked her to cross the road and grab a trolley. We were about 20 metres from a pedestrian crossing, but instead of walking to the crossing, she literally did what he said and ran straight across the road without looking left or right! It all happened so fast, I remember calling out at her and then seeing this bus coming straight for her – I let out the most blood-curdling scream (the other children hadn't noticed what had happened to Jess and were more concerned about me!)

The bus slammed on its brakes but from where I was, I couldn't tell if she had been hit or not. I was hysterical and just kept repeating, "Did it hit her? Did it hit her!" The bus had hit her and she was thrown three metres. Miraculously, (and thanks to her judo training) Jess walked away with just a graze on her back that hadn't even drawn blood! Someone who had seen the accident happen called an ambulance so Jess was checked over and given the all clear. However, an elderly lady on the bus – the person whom I think saved Jess's life when she saw Jess run into the road and screamed at the driver to stop – she went into shock and was taken to hospital. I never got to thank her, and I don't even know if she knew Jess was OK.

Jess's most recent battle with cancer has been her toughest challenge yet. My little miracle is still here to tell her story – and what an incredible story it is! I am so proud of you Jess; you are amazing. I love you to the moon and back, xxx

Heather – Jess's Mum

~ ~ ~

My parents made me feel like I had a normal childhood, for them it was filled with silent fears and they tried to wrap me in cotton wool, even while I was the most rebellious child you've ever met! I remember the endless bleeding of small cuts and bruises all over me that caused strangers to ask what Mummy and Daddy were doing to me! I remember making friends with kids my age who were really sick, because I was being treated in the oncology ward with them too. To think I was so unwell, we were offered a wish from Make A Wish Foundation! I could have gone to Disneyland if Mum hadn't turned it down – thanks Mum! She felt like it would be admitting defeat. Those years were challenging and confusing for me at such a young age, but the blessing of being able to now look it with a new lens allows me to see the strength and the skills I had started to develop at a young age.

I created an identity as a young, strong girl, who acknowledged her limitations but never let them hold her back; I still pushed the envelope. I learned to focus on what I had, and not on what I didn't; what I could do rather than what I couldn't. I continued to thrive. I got to learn new skills like cooking that I may never have learned if it wasn't for this experience, it's a passion I still have. But I think the most important for my future was realising that I didn't need to care about looking different and standing out. I got used to people staring and looking at me with my little white helmet with blue stars or making comments. It taught me to be comfortable with who I am.

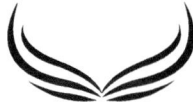

CHAPTER 16

THE SUNDANCE OF SPORT

*"It doesn't matter the size of the dog in the fight,
rather the size of the fight in the dog."*
— *Mark Twain*

Looking back, I can see how sport, specifically Judo, shaped my identity and revealed some inner strengths.

After moving to Australia, I became sports obsessed, trying out everything from ballet to basketball. One day when I was about ten, Mum decided to send my brother to try out Judo to help with his coordination. As soon as I heard that my ear pricked up and I begged to join him. Mum wasn't too sure on her uncoordinated ballerina joining a class of all boys doing martial arts but she said yes, thinking after one class I'd be sick of it, good golly how wrong she was!

I fell in love with the sport and the discipline. As a loud, dominant young leader I needed to learn the value in respect, determination, hard work and structure, all things required in Judo, along with at least trying to keep my loud mouth shut and listening to others. Within a year of consistent training I was competing at a state level! I felt so out of my depth at times. Judo seemed to be a family sport, most people got into it because of their parents and they had been doing it since they could walk. I on the other hand had no real training, I had been at it for a little while and only knew a handful of throws. However, what I did have was passion and drive!

There were very few females competing then so we were loped in with the males and split up into weight categories. With a sport that seemed boutique, especially in Melbourne, this meant that I had regular competition, and could measure my growth based upon my performance against consistent competitors. Starting to compete improved my skills, lessons turned into action, seeing what worked and learning by literally falling flat on my face, arse, back, side and every other section of my body that had some amount of surface area!

After a year of competing, I entered into the Victorian State Titles, at the time I thought it was just another competition but as I entered the hall, ready for weigh-in and the usual social banter, I could not have been more wrong! The whole energy of the room was focused, determined and regimented. It was extremely formal and stern; the usual laughter and enjoyment had dissipated and was replaced by pure determination. There were so many more people than I was used to seeing, so many unfamiliar faces. I felt a little alone and overwhelmed, I loved the social aspect of the competitions just as much as I loved the fighting itself, but that wasn't the aim of the day. The aim was to win and to qualify to represent Victoria at the Australian Championships.

I didn't really know if that was something I wanted but I did know that I was determined to win against some of my biggest competitors! As I moved my way through the line-up, winning round after round, sometimes by a lot and other times by the skin of my teeth. I was in the final, against one of my biggest competitors, Nick. He was strong, funny and let's be honest there was a little bit of harmless flirtation off the mat, on it however, I was going to come out on top. I did win, by the tiniest of throws and was given the honour of representing Victoria in the Australian championships the following year at the age of twelve.

I didn't really understand what that meant. I thought it would just be a similar competition, with lots of laughter and fun. But I quickly realised that wasn't the case, I was training on weekends with the top competitors in Victoria from all age groups, this wasn't the training I was used to; it was hard, gruelling and painful ... but I loved it! I was running every day. I was training extended hours at my usual Judo training, two and a half hours on a Wednesday and three hours a Sunday! It was crazy, I saw an elite sports mindset coach and she taught me to visualise winning before it had happened, visualise being on the number one spot and do everything I could to get there!

I dropped a weight group; I had my focus songs like, 'Eye of the Tiger' and 'Impi' (an African song about a white warrior.) I went from being a causal judo-goer who liked to socialise and enjoyed the sport to a determined fighter who was going to be the next Australian Champion.

In June 2006, I flew to Perth with my dad and judo gear in tow. Dad was always my number one Judo supporter, he was there on the sidelines cheering for everything, even at training. I was fresh meat and I had no clue what to expect, how hard the competition would be or even who it would be. I was surprised, and honestly a little disappointed that I would only be fighting against girls at this competition. I warmed up, I listened to my songs and I visualised myself standing on that podium with a gold medal in my hand. Most of the people around me seemed to be familiar with each other, like this wasn't their first time representing their state and mingling with competitors from other states.

For the first few rounds I realised I was being treated like the underdog with no experience, but after winning three rounds with a few big throws I felt like the attention was on me. Round after round I was winning and eventually to my delight ... and everyone else's surprise I was in the final. I felt like The Karate Kid, the opponent that nobody expected! My finals fight, I was against the favourite, I had watched her fight with passion and aggression, she knew she was the top dog and she would do anything to stay there! I knew there would be a lot of pushing, I figured out a few of her throws and that one of her tactics was to get foot fouls. I don't remember the actual fight, I just remember the pure focus and being announced the winner – only by the smallest of points. But I won!

Getting that medal, standing on that podium as number one proved to me that I could do anything I put my mind to, as long as I backed it up with hard work and determination. I felt on top of the world that day, I was a hero and I was so proud of myself!

Coming back home was really hard, my peers didn't know what Judo was and outside of the Judo world I got very little recognition. It was weird to go from being on top of the world and praised by my teammates to heading back to school and barely getting more than a 'nice job'. I felt like I had two lives, two personalities at times. There was the determined talkative leader at Judo who could be herself, have fun and didn't have to fit the mould of anything, I could be me. Then there was the schoolgirl Jess, who just wanted to be liked and accepted, who wanted to be recognised for her achievements but not at the risk of being labelled a weirdo. I became self-conscious of being a Judo player, because it was a rough sport. I wanted to be known for something else. I wanted to be normal too, have the boyfriend, have fun, go to parties and sometimes Judo seemed to get in the way of that.

The next year I competed again at the Nationals, this time it was held in Adelaide. I was one of the youngest in the under 16s age group and again a bit of an underdog but equally as determined. I placed first for the second year in a row! I had my sights set on competing forever and one day representing Australia in international competitions, maybe even the Olympics! I was now training three days a week, as well as running and building my fitness regime.

A few months after Nationals there was a call out for National team tryouts to go to the Australian Institute of Sport (AIS). The aim of this program was to get a team together for the 2012 Olympics which was about four years away. There was a minimum age of 15, I was a few months off that but was advised that if I placed well enough that would be waived. So I trained harder than ever before, this was my dream to get onto the team and I knew despite my age I could make it. The tryouts were half a day, we had crazy cardio testing, technique testing; it was exhilarating and draining. I was doing really well, the man in charge of choosing the team kept a close eye on me and I could tell he wanted me to get one of the spots.

Almost two hours in I was pulled aside and told I was too young and that I needed to step down. My heart shattered and I burst into tears, I was doing better than I could have ever imagined and this dream was being ripped out of my grasp regardless! I felt defeated as I left the tryouts, filled with anger and disappointment, not understanding why my age was such a barrier here.

Looking back, I know this was the moment when my passion started to slip, instead of pushing forward and above this I let it take its toll. Later that year, I had my second blow when I placed third at the National Championships in Sydney. I had gone up another weight group and hadn't realised the difference it would make, it was a whole new ball game! I left Sydney feeling crushed, wondering if I was good enough, strong enough or if I even had what it takes. I watched my friends who had been old enough to go to the AIS do incredibly well, the program had done wonders for them and it only made me more spiteful and angry.

I hadn't just let down myself, I had let down my family, my coach and the Victorian team, or so I thought. I let that burden hang over my head and instead of rising above it I let it crush me. I turned my focus to other things, like school, boys, partying and friendships. While I still found a haven on the judo mat I had also felt disconnected from it.

A year later, I was old enough to try out for the AIS Olympic team, I did try and I did well, but that desire burning in me the year before had dulled. I hadn't trained as hard, I wasn't as focused and it showed. I missed out on a scholarship spot that year but I was still offered the opportunity to pay my own way and go to train with the team, which I did and loved.

It was an incredible opportunity, and looking back I was still so young, I had so much working in my favour but that disappointment loomed over my head. Though it's an experience I will never ever forget, getting to compete and fight with the top athletes in Australia, looking back it's something I am so incredibly grateful for.

A few months later, while I was training hard, I had my fire back after realising how incredible being in the AIS team would be! I had trained with them and though I wasn't named in the "team" as such, my passion was burning.

One training session, I was practicing with one of my friends who was new to Judo. As she tried out a new throw, she put her arm out instead of landing properly and dislocated her elbow! I was overthrown with guilt as the ambulance was called. I was distraught and I wanted to call it quits for the night, my mind wasn't on the mat, it was with her and it was hard.

The trainers didn't want me to rest, they wanted to keep me moving, I had State Championships coming up and I needed all the practice I could get. During one training session, I stopped a throw being made on me, but then landed in such a way that I hyper-extended my knee. I was in agony and fell to the ground, knowing that this injury would set me back. My dreams were getting further and further away.

I was told I had to stay off the mat for eight weeks, which meant I couldn't compete in the Victorian State Championships and that I might not be able to qualify for Nationals. I felt like I was running on empty and decided it was time to take a step back to find my love and passion for Judo again. I needed to find myself and I wanted to have a year off from the pressure. I was 15, going into Year 10 at school and I just wanted time to relax and focus on me a little bit before I headed into my final years of schooling while training for the Olympics.

That decision didn't go down so well with my dad or my coach. They wanted me to push through but I started to push back. I have always been extremely stubborn. When my mind is made up, when I have set up my boundaries and my rules, I don't take well to being told I was wrong and making a mistake.

I had recognised I was burning out and wanted to save myself because I knew the love was there, but the timing wasn't right. I still managed to get accepted to represent Victoria in the Nationals even though I didn't compete, they based it on my merit from previous successful competitions.

I knew I hadn't trained much, my knee was giving me a lot of issues and I really wasn't in my best shape. I weighed just over the maximum in my weight group; only half a kilo over which was a little frustrating but I didn't view this as the end of the world for me; this was my year off, my year of fun. But I was the only one to see it like that; everyone else was devastated, stressed out and disappointed. On competition day, I tried to stay light-hearted while keeping my head in the game. The girls I were fighting where 7kgs heavier than me so I was at a disadvantage. One of the hardest things for me was that my dad wasn't there, this was our thing and he wasn't there. I had my loving mum by my side, and while she supported me, she didn't love seeing me on the mat, she sat there worried about me the whole time!

There were only three of us in my weight division including me, so with a small division, we had the opportunity to fight each other. I won the first round and in the second I was doing really well. I was smiling and laughing on the mat, enjoying myself. At one point my opponent fell and got a bloody nose. It took the medics a while to patch it up and while waited, I was light-heartedly dancing on the sidelines, still in my good mood. However, this break in the round caused me to lose focus on the competition. When the round recommenced, I found myself in a losing position very quickly.

I was disappointed, but it wasn't the end of the world, I had come to have fun, keep up practice and enjoy the competition. My coach though, was really upset with me. He said I had embarrassed him by not taking the competition seriously and dancing on the sidelines. I didn't see it from his side at the time; I was there to have fun. In my view, I was returning from an injury and in some ways, I was competing just to make him and my dad happy. It wasn't what I had wanted to do that year; I had said I wanted time out. In hindsight I understand his disappointment, it wasn't about losing, it was about the lack of respect I displayed to our sport.

I walked away from that competition irritated. I realised that my Judo world and 'normal' life outside of it were never going to blend; I couldn't have both. I would have to choose because neither of them would compromise for the other. I had to choose either the short-term goal of the Olympics that would hold me back in my long-term goal of studying and a career. I felt like I couldn't be an athlete and an academic, and at that point my love for the sport was gone and I was doing it for my coach and my dad, not for me. At the start of 2010 I just didn't return to Judo, the pressure and the constant feeling of sacrifice was too much for me.

After many years, I returned to Judo in 2014 and fell in love with the movement and the sport all over again. I wanted to compete again, just casually this time. The irony was that a few months later the cancer took it all away from me again. And after the brain surgery, I am no longer allowed to play contact sports.

Judo played such a pivotal part of my life growing up, channelling my drive, enabling me to set goals and focus my energy. Not only did Judo shape me and initiate me into the world of goals it also helped me tap into a new warrior attitude within.

Positive: Judo it was all about that positive mindset and knowing through and through that I can do this! Like many sports, if I got in my head, started focusing on what went wrong, what I did badly and gave those negative thought patterns any power, I had already lost. I discovered how the power of positive affirmations and language as a whole was incredibly important. Affirmations like, I am a champion. *I can do this. I am strong. I am a winner.* And then, using visualisations to embody the feeling of achieving my goals.

Adventure: the adventure was knowing that this wouldn't always be easy, but it was an opportunity to grow and learn from. It also took me on a journey of finding myself and my passions. I learned very quickly that each match and training was an opportunity to shine and learn. I started using empowering questions like: How can I improve? How can I achieve this goal? Who can I ask for help?"

And to avoid disempowering questions like, "why do I always lose?" or "why am I not good enough?"

Thankful: I was grateful that I got these experiences, I was taught to be independent, resourceful, resilient and disciplined. To stick to my dreams when it gets tough because I never know what's on the other side. I am also grateful I found a community that accepted me as I was, and loved me for it. I always felt like I could be my authentic self at judo and that was amazing when I didn't feel like that out in the real world or at school.

Create: I created massive goals, and learned to set them in a way that kept me motivated and excited! To have grit, to keep going when my body was sore, or I was tired. To have a strong reason why and to utilise visualisations to help me connect to the gratification of achieving my goals.

Honour: I honoured myself by believing in my capabilities, by being my own cheerleader and being proud of my achievements and by listening to my needs, setting boundaries and knowing when it was time for me to walk away.

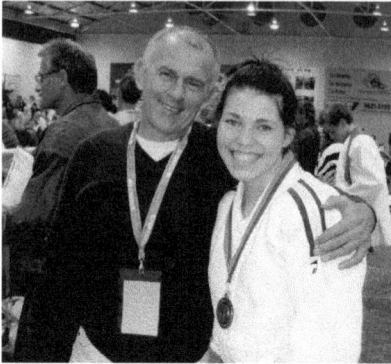
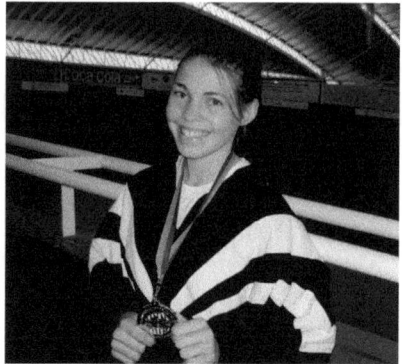
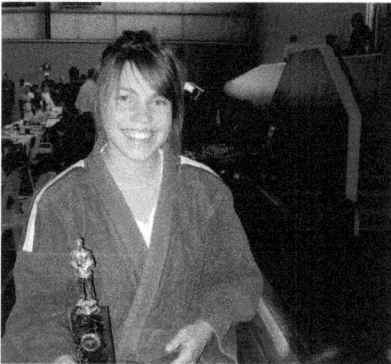
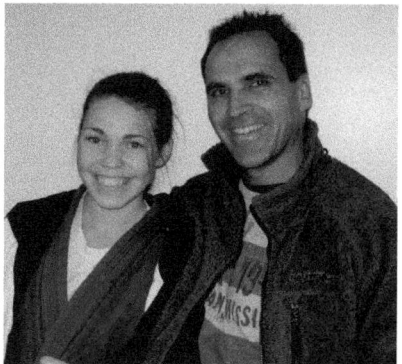
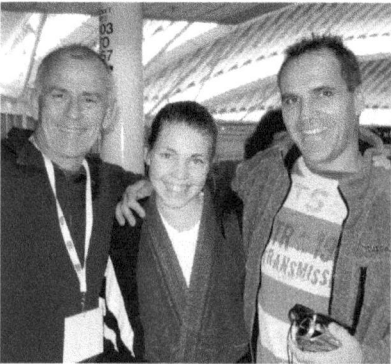
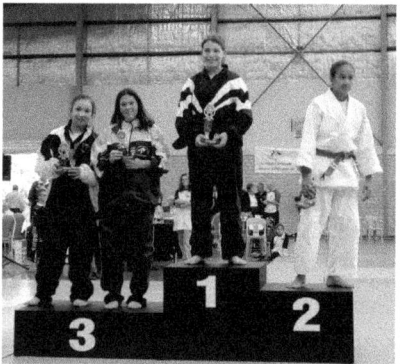

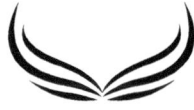

CHAPTER 17

THE SUNDANCE BETWEEN LOVE AND FEAR

"We may not be able to prepare the future for our children, but we can at least prepare our children for the future."
— *President Franklin D. Roosevelt*

I was blessed (although at the time it felt burdened) with three younger siblings within a short space of time. When I was three years old, Mum fell pregnant with twins. I remember helping to choose names and decorate their rooms. When Mum became quite unwell and was admitted to hospital, I was happy to stay with my Granny Arlene and Grandpa Tumble for a few days. They doted on me like a doll and I loved their three fluffy cats. Grandpa would give me all the chocolate shortbread tumbles I wanted, hence his nickname.

I remember a few days later, Granny handed me the phone. *"You're a big sister now Jessie!"* I was so excited to meet my little brother and sister; twins! I had to wait a few more days to visit my parents; the twins had arrived a month early and Mum was still very unwell.

Having siblings quickly lost its glamour when I realised I was no longer an only child and these two babies could only cry, poop and sleep. They were boring and to make it worse they got all the attention, my attention and I was missing it! At one point I asked my mum if could send the babies back.

To make things worse, a short five months later, Mum told me I was getting another baby. I was not happy! These twins had ruined my life already, and now there was going to be another one! After the shock and a few tantrums later I decided if Brittany and Daniel got to be twins and room buddies, then the new baby would be my twin; we would share a room and she would be my best friend and twin forever.

When Amy was born life changed a lot! Not only did we have another screaming baby in the house, but Dad was travelling overseas for work more than ever before. Granny Annie moved into our cottage out the back to help look after the babies. The twins were not sleeping at all, Amy slept in Granny's flat and she would feed her overnight to help ease the strain on my mum. She was solo parenting four children under five for the most part! She had my granny, our live-in nanny, Dora, and a cleaner to help take away some of the pressure off, but I don't think it ever did.

I remember one day standing next to the pool with Mum and getting very upset and confused as to where my dad was and why he was away so much. I remember looking up at her with the biggest pout on my face and said with innocence, *"Why is Daddy always on holidays?"* Mum was taken aback by this question, she struggled to answer, *"He's not on holidays, he's away for work, he loves you."* As I grew older I learned there was only one truth in that sentence; that he loves me.

The truth was that my dad had been overwhelmed with the idea of four children and had begun an affair with a woman he worked with. When Amy was born he left and started living with the woman he had been seeing, it was the reason my dad was away so much and why my granny moved in. Although I didn't know the details, I always knew something was wrong; I was worried, I was hurt and I felt alone. I had been a Daddy's girl and the centre of my parents' world, as soon as my siblings arrived, my life fell apart and I didn't like all this change and probably blamed them for it! My mum tried to keep me distracted, she knew I found it hard and I was probably the first child in recorded history to have a four-and-a-half-year-old birthday party. I felt like a princess even though Mum told my friends no presents!

After a while Dad came back home and I settled into life as a sister and 'twin' to Amy who was four and a half years younger than me. I was the big girl, learning to change nappies when I was five and I came to love looking after my siblings.

Dad was more present and although he still (actually) travelled for work he was never gone for as long. As a family we moved to Australia in 2002 and a few years later my parents renewed their wedding vows, we were a solid loving family unit. We did everything together; my parents were incredibly affectionate with each other (I thought it was gross at ten years old) and with us. It seemed to everyone including my mum that the behaviours that had been breaking down their marriage in South Africa were behind them.

However, when I was 13 years old, I heard Mum and Dad having an incredibly explosive fight over the phone while Dad was overseas for work. Mum was screaming, *"How could you do this to me again!"* Her shrill voice was breaking painfully between words, a sound that sent shivers down my spine and hit me in the chest; it was a sound of pain, betrayal and torture. I couldn't hear Dad's answer, just another sob from Mum a few minutes later, *"You're having an affair Craig!"* She sounded like a woman lost and defeated.

I had never heard her sound like that and I wanted to race in and hug her, but I felt like it wasn't my place, they were the adults, they'd sort it out – hopefully. I knocked on Mum's door later to find her still crying; she looked so empty. I hugged her, *"Are you going to get a divorce?"*

She held me close, *"I am so sorry my Jess, what did you hear?"*

I gulped, I didn't want her to think I had been spying on them, *"That Dad's having an affair, does that mean he's cheating on you?"* Mum just silently sobbed, she knew that in that moment I had lost so much of my childhood innocence, that I was being dragged into an adult life before I was ready or could even comprehend it.

"Yes. But it was just once and it's over, we will sort this out Jess, I promise." And my heart broke, my dad, my idol, the man of my life had just broken my trust.

~ Pretending to Parent ~

Mum usually loved to wake us up each morning with a cup of tea and a huge smile. *"Wake up, wake up, it's a lovely day,"* she would sing extremely out of tune. The next day however, she was nowhere to be seen and I realised she'd stayed in bed. I took it upon myself to wake up my siblings and get them ready for school. I knew how hurt I was and I wanted to protect them from that same pain and distrust, they were too young to know what I knew.

The next day was the same. My brother and sister started to ask questions but I wanted to shelter them, *"It's OK, Mum is just a bit sick at the moment and she's asked me to get you ready and she'll take us down to school."*

Mum stayed in this state for about a week, I felt like a step-in mum. I didn't let my siblings bother her, I helped cook and didn't complain when I couldn't make it to Judo that week. My granny was around a lot that week too and together we took up the slack so that Mum could pick herself back up.

When Dad came back from his work trip I felt angry and irritated with him, but also a little relieved because I didn't want my parents to break up. I couldn't bring myself to talk to him for a while.

I was incredibly independent at that stage and once he was home I was out of sight, avoiding him at all costs yet sending him incredibly angry text messages, calling him an asshole among many other things. I couldn't believe that he was just back in our house as if nothing had happened. I didn't get it. That was the moment I took on the role as my mum's protector and being an adult figure and source of stability to my siblings.

I kept what I knew hidden for years. It was so lonely at times; I had no one to talk to because my siblings didn't know. Only I could see the patterns, the deep lows of sadness and depression that would take over Mum. I could read the signs, the longer than usual work trips or unexpected delays, the lying, the fighting, the frustration, the weight loss, the snide comments and the silence. I would pull my siblings away at any sign of distress and put on a movie or play outside. I still hoped my parents would work it out but thought my siblings were too young to go through this, I didn't think they'd understand.

The hardest thing was feeling like I had to pick sides, what my dad was doing was morally wrong in my eyes. I hated that, but he was still my dad and I still loved him! I started to believe that the affair was about more than my parents, wondering why our family wasn't enough for my dad, wondering what we could do to make him stay. We had such amazing times as a family, so many beautiful holidays and weekends together that I couldn't comprehend it.

Later that year Dad brought along a woman – another 'work friend' – to one of my judo competitions. I don't believe he knew then, that I knew the affair was still going on. But when he introduced us, I lost concentration. I became plagued with thoughts of losing "our thing" – as Judo was always something we did together, I didn't want to lose it. I didn't want to lose him.

The affair continued on and off, perhaps for a few years. It wasn't until I was in Year 9 and about to turn 15 that everything seemed to escalate. My parents seemed on rockier ground than ever before; there didn't seem to be an in-between to passionately in love or devastated and heartbroken, it was a yo-yo of emotions that was hard to keep up with. Eventually it got so bad he left, and moved in with the woman he was seeing. My siblings were so confused, he had been overseas for work and when he came back he moved straight in with HER. They felt blindsided and in shock, as I explained to them what was going on. They were now about the same age as when I found out and while it wasn't ideal, I felt like I had done the best I could to shelter them for as long as possible.

In the months to come Dad would ask us to go and stay at his house, which caused a rift in our sibling relationship. While Amy and Daniel wanted to maintain their relationship with Dad and spend time with him, Brittany and I refused to be anywhere near 'that homewrecker's house'. In my mind Amy and Dan were wrong and betraying Mum. In reality, it was just that they weren't following my beliefs, it was a tough situation to be in and both choices were tough.

I got incredibly sick at this point. I wasn't able to eat, I was running fevers and with glandular fever going around school I thought it could be that. Multiple tests later though I was told it was stress sickness, I was literally worried sick about my mum, my siblings and what the future had in store for us all.

In some ways it was a relief that my siblings knew what was going on, I didn't feel so alone and they were people who were going through this with me. I didn't really have anyone outside of my family to talk to. I didn't want to be a 'debbie downer' or a burden so I learned to keep it close to my chest and let it out by journaling or through Judo.

I was very confused to find out about five months later, he had moved out of HER house and in with a friend. Mum decided she wouldn't just let him move back in, he would need to prove that he was well and truly done with it all. Which he did, and after a few more months he moved back in with us. I so vividly remember my dad sitting us down and crying and apologising for everything he had done. He said he'd learnt his lesson that, 'the grass wasn't always greener on the other side, instead of crossing every bridge in sight when things get tough he should stick around and water his own grass.'

~ Wild and Trapped ~

I mistrusted him and still felt hurt; I began to spend more and more time away from home. I became rebellious, knowing that if my dad, 'the rule maker' didn't have to follow the rules – why should I? I tested every boundary, and was grounded regularly ... not that I took that punishment seriously either.

I also vowed to never get myself into my mum's situation. I judged her for staying, for sticking it out, for putting up with the crap. I labelled that kind of love and forgiveness as weak and promised myself I would never be dependent on anyone else like that. I would never let a man get so close to me that he could hurt me and I would never forgive a man the way she did. I was too naive to understand the emotional attachment between them, never having been in love myself at that point. I have also since realised how strong Mum was in finding forgiveness for him. She did it for her own sake but also for our whole family, she wanted to keep us together and give us a stable loving home. I now see the reason why she stayed is because Mum took her wedding vows 'till-death-do-us-part' seriously. She never wanted us to have a broken home. She did everything she could so that wouldn't happen, include sacrifice herself.

When he came home we were already on our annual family holiday in Merimbula, a beautiful beachside town in NSW, which had glorious beaches and felt a million miles away from everything. Soon after he flew in to join us, I knew something was off. Within a few days I found out it was much more than that. I had borrowed his laptop to do the typical pre-smartphone, Facebook-check and as I was sitting there I heard the familiar sound of a Skype message come through, my heart sank as I saw HER name, knowing my dad was up to his same old crap.

I felt so trapped. I didn't want to tell Mum and be the person to ruin our holidays.

I wore the burden as if it were my own to carry, as if it would be my fault if the trip were ruined. I didn't know what to do; it felt like a lose-lose situation. I knew Mum would just forgive him anyway so what was the point in causing drama over something when I knew how it would end. I was grateful to have other family friends around that I could escape to. I couldn't tell them what was going on in my parents' private lives but they did distract me from having to deal with it. I also didn't want my dad to think I was spying on him or taking my mum's side. It was such a difficult time to navigate, I didn't want to get into a confrontation, I was looking for ways to reduce the pressure on me.

When we returned home my rebellious streak continued, I spent even less time at home and got myself into a few situations where way too much alcohol was involved. It got to the point where my parents lifted all the rules realising that the rules were guiding my rebellion. They said I was an adult and adults have to deal with the consequences of their actions. They said they would be there to guide me but ultimately, I had to make my decisions and wear the consequences, whatever they were. No more grounding, no more confiscating of phones and laptops. They laid down three rules in stone: no sleepovers with boys; no going out on school nights, and finally if I found myself in trouble, no matter how late or how far away, I could call them no questions asked.

This worked for me, it gave me freedom, I was being recognised as an adult and I knew those three rules were in place for a reason not 'just because they said', so I stuck to them. I still avoided home every weekend I could. Sometimes I felt guilty for leaving my siblings to deal with the fragile environment at home, but I also felt helpless and that it wasn't my job to be there and support them the whole time, I wanted to live my teenage years on my terms, not as a second mum to my siblings. This was an internal debate I would have with myself for years.

During our family trip back to South Africa, my parents had seemed on a high yet the shit hit the fan when Dad moved out just a few months later! After he moved into HER house for the second time, I stepped straight back into the role of second parent at home. I remember my friends at school bringing me chocolate and trying to console me the best they could. It was something that I appreciated but also felt incredibly uneasy about, I didn't want people to know what was going on at home, I didn't want them to know that I was struggling. For a few weeks they would check in on me but as time passed and life kept moving it was no longer a hot topic.

My anger towards my dad grew stronger as I looked at his betrayal for the second time, trying to make sense of it. I wanted to protect my family but I also just wanted a normal life, I didn't want to have to worry about my mum, my siblings, my lifestyle and I resented him for taking that away from me.

I avoided seeing him over this period, I was aloof but also made it very clear I would not make time to fit him into my life. I watched as the cycle took its usual path. Six months after moving out of our family home and into HER house he was ready to come back home. Again, he moved in with a friend for three months and next thing I knew he was back in our home making the same speech about, 'the grass isn't greener...'

I was furious that Mum had taken him back again, that he was being forgiven for everything and there were no repercussions. I became more and more independent in an attempt to run away from the problems at home, relying on my friends and my boyfriend to be there and provide stability.

With time those feelings settled, although I didn't trust my dad I did love him and hated being angry at him; I missed having a relationship with him. Shortly after he came back home, his mum Granny Arlene, passed away and he flew to South Africa to organise everything. It was weird because I had just opened up to him and then he disappeared again and I didn't know what to make of it

The next year Dad's focus shifted, he had lost his mum and then his stepfather Grandpa Tumble was incredibly sick so he started to spend a lot of time back in South Africa. In 2010 he spent five months there. Time apart seemed to bring my parents closer together at first. But then Mum stopped working in order to renovate our family home ready for sale. This brought up a lot of resentment and expectations that I didn't understand. I felt like my dad's respect for my mum had disappeared. No matter what she did, it was never enough, she was 'spending too much', not getting renovations done 'fast enough', they weren't 'good enough', the house wasn't valued 'high enough'.

My mum started shrinking more and more into herself, feeling helpless, worthless even. I wanted to shake her, to tell her to be stronger, for her to realise that this wasn't healthy. Yet when Dad was home she seemed happy, it still seemed to lift her, give her purpose. On top of that I used to still periodically find out that Dad was still talking to HER. I didn't know whether they were still seeing each other or if it was an emotional affair, but it pushed me away and I lost a lot of respect for both of my parents.

~ Shifting Sands ~

Later in 2010, I booked a trip to South Africa, to visit my grandpa for what may be the last time and spend some time travelling. Dad had also started a business there to try and make ends meet while he was spending so much time over there. It was a big trip emotionally, spending so much time one-on-one with my dad in some ways made me miss that relationship we used to have and crave his presence in my life. It also made me resent him for letting everything get in the way of it.

Grandpa Tumble had Alzheimer's and was declining quickly. I went to the neurologist with him one day and it was so difficult to watch this incredibly bright man unable to draw a clock. Meanwhile my Grandpa Allen (Dad's biological dad) was fighting fit and still working full time! This trip taught me a lot; that I could have a relationship with my dad that wasn't necessarily a typical parental relationship, but it was a close friendship, and also that I could let go of some of that emotional attachment and ache for my parents to be together.

As Dad's business got bigger and Grandpa became sicker, Dad was home less and less. In 2011 when I was in Year 12, he was home for three months of the year total! I struggled to understand how my parents were still together with such little physical time together and while there was talk of a move at some point I didn't know what that would look like. I was so focused on getting through Year 12 and maintaining my relationship with my boyfriend and friends that I didn't even take notice of what was happening, emotionally detached in many ways.

Not having my dad there through my final year of school was hard; I didn't have stability or consistency at home. The shifts and swings of my parents' relationship felt like Groundhog day, the patterns were the same and my emotional responses followed the same cycle. I disengaged a lot of the time, finding it easier to have no expectations of Dad or the rest of my family. That harbouring of emotions was exhausting, and used to end in fiery explosions of anger, slamming doors or locking myself away in my room.

I couldn't emotionally invest in their relationship because I didn't believe it would continue to stay in this happy place for long. I focused on my future, planning to travel the year after school and then move out shortly after. I wanted and needed that distance, to feel like I could live my own life rather than putting out spot fires in everyone else's.

In March 2012, I left home to travel the world with my boyfriend, living with his family at times or in European backpackers, working in London and loving life. We planned to finish off our travels in South Africa where Mum and Dad would join us. While I was on this amazing trip Dad was still spending the majority of his time in South Africa, but his relationship with my mum and my siblings seemed to be growing stronger every time I spoke to them. In May, we met Dad in Belgium for a family friend's wedding, it was beautiful and fun sharing the experience with him. I felt at ease and after the crazy few months of travelling it was nice to have a piece of home with me.

One night I went to use dad's laptop to Skype home to talk to my mum. I fell into an old habit of snooping and mistrust when I saw HER name on his Skype account and went looking for their interactions. To my surprise I saw nothing, no conversations, no calls. I was still doubtful but wanted to think maybe things really had changed! Then as I sat there waiting for my call to go through, I heard the Skype notification noise go off, and my heart sank once again to see HER name lighting up. I clicked on it to see, 'Hey babe', written right there in front of me and I knew it wasn't over. The lies had continued and I was so torn, part of me didn't want to care, it's not my place, this is my parents' relationship and Mum was the one that kept letting him back in. The other part was the protective side of me that wanted to throw his laptop against a wall and tell him to fuck right off with his deception and utter bullshit.

I decided to ignore it; I wanted to enjoy my time with my dad at the end of the day. It was so hard with anger and mistrust boiling beneath my skin. I was fiery, short-tempered and closed off because I hadn't forgiven him, or forgotten those feelings I'd swept under the rug. I wrestled with my reactions, knowing I had lost even more respect for my dad this time, but also that I had been wrong to have given him the benefit of the doubt about turning his life around; when I saw that message, I felt like a fool for ever believing him.

It was still hard to say goodbye to my dad, seeing him had relieved a lot of the loneliness I'd felt while travelling but knowing things at home had not changed made me reluctant to go home too. For the rest of my time in Europe I was distanced from my dad and my family. I didn't want to call home as often because I was torn up inside about not telling Mum what I had seen. I felt like I had the world on my shoulders even from half way around the world, and the only way to escape that feeling was to avoid my family all together.

When I reached South Africa in the November, I had mixed feelings about seeing my parents. On one hand I was so excited to have them. I had been missing them like crazy and had felt so alone and trapped in my relationship with my boyfriend that I couldn't wait to get some distance and some perspective. On the other hand, I felt awkward around them; I knew I was keeping a secret. I could see how happy they seemed but also how fragile that happiness was. I didn't want to put a foot wrong and ruin their relationship.

My mum was only in South Africa for a few weeks and while she was there I saw my parents come together as a unit. While I was still sceptical, there was also the little girl inside me who wanted to believe they could still turn it around. Saying goodbye to Mum was the hardest thing, I still had two months ahead of me of incredible travel plans but my relationship with my boyfriend was on the rocks and I really needed my mum. I wanted to keep experiencing the world but I didn't want to do it in the relationship I was in.

Soon after she left we said goodbye to my dad too, we wouldn't see him until a week before we left to head back to Melbourne. My parents still tried to call every day while we were travelling. I know they were worried but I felt trapped by them and by my own relationship that was falling apart. I didn't feel strong enough to rebel against my relationship so I just rebelled against them, avoiding their calls for days on end. I was still so confused by the relationship my dad seemed to be putting on with my mum, I know she believed it, and I would have too, if I hadn't seen those messages in Belgium.

My parents were angry with me as they were terrified about our safety travelling around South Africa. The threat of kidnapping, muggings, rape and murder were all very real in one of the world's most dangerous countries. But I didn't care because I was hurting too. I didn't know how to communicate with them other than not communicating. There were so many bullets to dodge in a conversation that it was easier to stay quiet.

When I met up with my dad again, there was a lot more pent-up anger on both sides. He was angry at me for not communicating and taking his calls every day. While I had been brooding on everything that had happened with my parents and dreaded moving back home and having to live through it all again. But we calmed down fairly quickly and when it was time to leave I wasn't ready to go home to Melbourne.

~ Life Moves On ~

Getting home was disastrous; I didn't know where I fitted in with my family, socially or with work. A year abroad had turned everything on its head for me and life had moved on from when I left. My siblings had grown up so much and created a really strong bond; one I didn't fit into. I felt distanced from my mum because I didn't know what I could or should say to her about my dad. My friends had all started uni or work and with a lot of them it felt like we were on different pages. I struggled to find work having come home just as the busy summer was ending. On top of that my relationship with my boyfriend was breaking down before my eyes. I had to create my life from the ground up and it was tough but I got there.

A few months later Dad came to home to visit and I knew something was really off. Mum and him were jarring again, harder than ever and fighting more often and more openly than ever before. Dad was angry, perpetually, and it seemed to trickle into every interaction he had. He started huge fights with everyone, and even yelled at people he didn't know. One interaction I will never forget. As we sat around the dinner table Dad was telling a story about an interaction he had had that day with a person who hit his car with their hands as they crossed in front of it, it ended with him yelling, *"Don't you fucking dare hit my car, who the fuck do you think you are?!"*

My siblings and I all looked very confronted and confused, we had been brought up not to swear and now Dad was dropping the f-bomb over dinner. Mum wasn't impressed either and told him not to swear in front of us. The fight escalated as Dad had decided we were old enough to hear a swear word or two but Mum didn't agree. The yelling grew louder and ended as Dad yelled, *"Fuck you!"* straight to her face and stormed off. The entire table was in shock, my mum's eyes glazed over with tears and my heart broke as I made my decision; this had gone too far and I was done sitting on the sidelines!

The next day I told my dad point blank, *"If you aren't happy in this marriage then you need to leave. I cannot watch you treat my mum like that and I can see you are miserable. Right now, you are not being a good role model to any of us, and while I can see that, I don't know if my siblings can. You are showing my sisters that it's OK to be treated like that by a man. And you are showing my brother that it's OK to treat a woman and his future wife the way you have been treating my mum and it's not!"* I don't know what I thought would come of it; I just wanted everyone to stop being hurt and the only way I saw that happening was by something significantly changing. I don't know if I thought he would leave, just that it might jolt him into changing his ways.

A few days later my parents sat us all down and announced that they were separating; Dad was moving back to South Africa permanently. He had recognised that he needed to find himself again and said he didn't feel he could do that while trying to fix everything else. My siblings cried, begging him to stay, Mum looked heartbroken and I yelled out, *"No! Don't do this!"* I was furious at myself and at him.

I felt that I was the reason he was leaving, that he was using my conversation with him as permission. I blamed myself, and it felt like a load of bricks falling on top of me. I wished I had never opened my mouth when I saw the devastation that washed over the room. My moment of brash, honest and blunt opinions had just impacted my whole family and torn them apart. I was sick to my stomach; feeling like the worst sister and daughter in the world, I had meddled in business that wasn't mine.

~ Unravelling ~

We all went through the stages of grief at different times, from denial, anger, bargaining, depression and acceptance. I tried to still be the strength for my family, but I struggled to do so. I blamed myself for every emotion they had, every worry, every tear, while I managed to stay strong on the outside on the inside I was eroding. I didn't know how to stay strong but I also didn't know how to communicate that I wasn't strong; I leant back on my habits of avoidance. I spent time surrounded by friends, partying, working, studying and ignoring the real problems. I pretended I was fine as I latched onto my friendships. My self-blame came out as anger and being short tempered at home, my room was a mess that replicated my headspace.

Our home life was weird. I was still trying to find my place at home and my family was scattered trying to deal with the new changes that we faced.

Mum blamed Dad for leaving and causing such distress for my siblings. But because I blamed myself and took responsibility for my dad leaving, all I heard was, *"This is your fault,"* and I slumped lower and lower. I tried to stay bubbly Jess on the outside but inside it was dark, I wondered whether anyone would miss me if I was gone, I wondered if life would be better for the people around me if I wasn't here. I thought about moving away, I thought about leaving, I thought I was worthless and all I caused was drama.

When Dad came back to visit I started to experience anxiety, I felt so much pressure to make the most of the time with him, while I still tried to maintain my busy lifestyle, make Mum feel loved and everything else.

The first time I had a full-blown anxiety attack was at work. My dad had missed his flight and the next one he could get wasn't for a few days, with exam periods coming up it meant I had lost the days I had planned to spend with him. I was mad at him, I believed if our plans were that important to him he would have made his flight and now he just expected me to rearrange my week and my time to suit him even though I was at my wits' end with university and work.

He came into the busy café where I worked to try and spend time with me, trying to talk to me while I was busy keeping all my customers happy. I remember saying to my best friend Alanna, who worked with me, that I couldn't breathe, that I felt trapped, that my heart was racing and my head was spinning, I felt hot and clammy, that I just wanted to sit on the floor and crawl up into a ball. She knew these were signs of anxiety and told me to take a break and get some fresh air. I didn't listen, I could see my section getting busier and I wanted to keep working, but a few moments later I was so overwhelmed I was running for the bathroom unable to breath, tears streaming down my face and panicking through the roof!

I still didn't know what was going on, I didn't have anxiety – only people who had been diagnosed with anxiety could have anxiety attacks! But my laboured breaths and heavy chest suggested otherwise. Alanna had seen my mad dash for the bathroom and thankfully followed me and took charge of the situation. She broke the attack, talked me through slowing my breaths down even as I cried, *"It's too much, it's all too much, I can't work and deal with my dad, I just can't, it's too much!"* I didn't know how else to articulate it, I didn't know what else to say because I had been holding in so much anger, had suppressed so much of what had happened over the years that it burst out of me and I was terrified!

Once I was calm enough to be left alone, Alanna went out and told my dad he needed to leave, that I wasn't ready to see him. She told my boss I had an anxiety attack and needed to go home. I called Mum and told her I had an anxiety attack. I felt so weird, not recognising myself anymore with so much anxiety, self-doubt and deep-seated blame. It was a result of not confronting my emotions but rather bottling them up hoping they would go away and then being terrified when they were about to explode out of me.

The anxiety attack was terrifying and a real wake-up call. I needed to set boundaries for myself and my relationships; especially with my dad. I knew he wanted to feel connected and involved in my life but I wasn't ready for that. I needed to deal with where I was emotionally, and to understand what I expected from our relationship. It was a chance to create our relationship from the ground up which felt like both a blessing and a curse.

I needed to stand my ground and realise that at this point I was an adult and respect was a two-way street that is earned, not freely given. Finding this balance took time and a lot of work! There were weeks, sometimes months, where I didn't speak to my dad as we tried to define our father-daughter relationship. It's something that didn't happen overnight that's for sure.

~ Common Ground ~

It was later that year that I would hear 'cancer' for the first time. It put a lot of those questions of self-worth and emotions to rest. It took facing my own mortality to realise that I was loved, that I was appreciated, but more than that it made me realise how much I valued life and every single day being a blessing. That scare was a wakeup call to stop being so caught up in the drama, to realise that I had so much to offer and realise that I needed to appreciate every day and not hold onto the past. Now I know that can be easier said than done, but this was the first step in the right direction. My parents really came together during this time, looking after me as a team and I thought this would unite them as friends, create a foundation for a strong co-parenting relationship.

That wasn't the case, the next year my parents seemed to fight more than they ever had when they were together. There was so much anger on both sides and it often felt like me and my siblings were the pawns in the middle. As the year went on I was still trying to figure out what I wanted my relationship to look like with Dad and there were decisions I made with the pure desire to avoid drama. With my 21st birthday, I decided not to invite my dad, knowing that he and my mum couldn't stand to be in a room together. I was happy with this decision, especially when my dad wanted to stop Mum coming out for dinner with us on my actual birthday. I put my foot down, saying that wasn't happening and if she didn't come I would cancel the booking (look at those boundaries in action!). But that night, they actually got along for the first time in a long time. I was feeling relaxed around my dad and I began to regret my decision not to invite him. I felt terrible, that I had let him down and myself; I begged him to change his flight, to stay and be here for my 21st but it was too late for that. I had made a decision and I had to accept the consequences.

One day, Mum opened up to me by saying, *"I wish he didn't leave!"* With tears in her eyes she said, *"It's so hard to know he chose to leave me and our life behind, he has ruined everything."*

I burst out and said, *"I'm sorry, I'm sorry, I'm sorry! I told him to leave! It's my fault, I did it, but you can't keep blaming me! I did what I thought was best at the time and I get it, I fucked up and I ruined your life but you can't keep blaming me for it!"*

I wept and Mum looked shocked, *"Jess, he is an adult, he chose to leave. I don't blame you and I've never blamed you. I know it was the right thing, I just wish it didn't end this way."*

My mum held me close and for the first time in almost two years I let go of the blame I had been holding onto, the self-deprecation and hate that was crippling me. I realised I didn't have the control to make him leave, that was all him. I felt free, from a burden I didn't realise I was carrying until that point. I didn't realise I was blaming myself so wholeheartedly, I didn't realise I had thought everyone else blamed me.

My relationship with my dad continued to be rocky for years as we learned to create the foundations of our new relationship. There were loads of ups and special memories we shared like being in South Africa together. There were hard times like being diagnosed, having to fundraise, having to learn to support each other and my family together as a unit. There have been downs where we didn't talk for months on end due to disagreements or boundaries being breached. It's taken a lot of work, communication, understanding and forgiveness to create the relationship we have now but it has all been worth it.

Recently, I had the most profound conversation with my dad, it was open, honest and raw. It was the first time I felt like we were equals and I was getting to see the real man behind the mask, a mask I didn't know he was wearing, but there was also a woman hiding behind my mask. We both thought we had to show up as, 'other people' to our relationship. Dad had always tried to be strong and all knowing, while I had been young and timid. I acted like 16-year-old Jess and in return I was treated that way, it was a cycle that had to be broken, our behaviours had to change.

The conversation started by me thanking him for all the lessons I had learned from him. I was strong, independent, capable and stubborn. So much of who I am today is thanks to him, as well as some of the hardship from my parents' marriage breakdown, and although it was hard, I am grateful.

Then I listened as he told me his version of the events. They didn't paint him as a hero, they painted a man who was stuck, *"I felt lost as I looked back on my life. I was so far off the path from the man I used to be, a man who had strong values. I hated where I was, how I was acting, who I was being, it didn't feel right but I didn't know how to change. I felt at that point I was not being a good role model for you, any of you. I wasn't proud of the man I was and I knew I needed to find myself again, but between the travelling back and forth to South Africa and the stress of a failing marriage I didn't feel like I had another option than to cut it off and find myself."* He spoke with tears in his eyes and I finally felt like I could see him and the pain that he has been through. I felt a deep level of respect for him being so open with me and it rekindled my trust in him.

I learned to forgive him but also ask for forgiveness. I learned to appreciate all the lessons I learned through this journey. I learned to communicate, openly, honestly and fully. I learned to set boundaries for myself and what I will and will not accept.

His open vulnerability allowed me to see the real man. I was always a Daddy's girl growing up, I used to idolise him, I thought he was the bee's knees and I wanted his approval and love more than anything. As I grew up that never changed, I knew he liked that I was strong-willed, determined, stubborn, strong, emotionally stable and a leader. While they are all characteristics that are a part of me, they aren't all of me. But it's who I felt I needed to be in order to be loved, not just by my dad but by anyone. I could understand him needing to find himself, in wanting to become a better person.

I've also had the pleasure of watching Mum grow so much since she was no longer being pulled down and criticised. I have watched her find her confidence, self-love and insane amounts of sass! When anyone is belittled or made to feel unworthy they learn to hide themselves from the world in fear of not being accepted by anyone else.

My role in the story of my parents' marriage has been one of the hardest, most formative experiences of my life. My lessons and growth from this long period can be summed up in PATCH below and I hope you will apply this method for finding resilience and success through your own hardship.

Positive: There is a difference between burying "negative" emotions to only focus on the positive ones and choosing to live in a powerfully positive state. The first is avoidance, it can cause outbursts, anxiety and numbness while the other is a choice to experience all emotions, they all have their place but give power to the emotional states you choose to live in.

Adventure: the adventure was finding my voice. Knowing that I could stand up for what I believe in. It's been an adventure that has united my family and created a strong bond with my siblings, with my mum and most recently my dad.

Thankful: I am grateful for this experience, writing that is making me cry. It's true but hard to say out loud because I know how much pain this journey has caused. Its taught me to be strong, to stand for what I believe in, that family is everything, to keep moving forward. It taught me lessons of what not to do in a relationship, how not to communicate, how not to act. It taught me what a toxic relationship looks like and can feel like so that I could recognise that on my own.

Create: I learned to create boundaries, how I choose to accept to be spoken to as well as treated, learning to say no and choosing where I want to spend my energy. Boundaries are based around my values and also around my own self-awareness, what do I need, how does this make me feel, what do I want. This is hard at times, I started off feeling guilty and selfish, but realised with time that these boundaries were important for me to maintain my integrity, to fill my own cup and actually build strong relationships rather than feeling resentment.

Honour: honouring myself, boundaries come into this. But also learning to have a voice and stand for what I believe in. This was hard with my parents, because growing up I always believed they had the final say, they were wise they guided me, so to then have that turn and realise that I didn't always agree with what they were saying and doing acting was tough but it taught me I have a right to use my voice, to express how I am feeling and that if I wish to see change being made it's up to me!

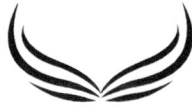

CHAPTER 18

THE DANCE OF FIRST LOVE:
HE LOVES ME, HE LOVES ME NOT

"The giving of love is an education in itself."
— *Eleanor Roosevelt*

I met Ben when I was 15 years old, at a small concert on the Mornington Peninsula, we had a few friends in common and had connected immediately. He was a tall blonde-haired surfer boy that I had this magnetic chemistry with, he was a gentleman and I wanted to know more. The next time we met was at midnight on my street, my friend and I sneaked out of home. Ben and his friends had also snuck out, and then walked over 4km to meet us out the front of my house. It was innocent fun, we walked, talked and laughed the whole time; we were in our own little bubble. He kissed me and I was hooked. We spent hours texting or on the phone because he lived almost an hour away by bus. I enjoyed his company and he treated me like a princess.

I opened up to him about my dad and told him my biggest fear was to trust someone and to get hurt, that I was scared he would be just like my dad. He responded, *"I promise I will never ever do what your dad has done. You're perfect and all I will ever need."* My heart skipped a beat and I started to let him in, trusting him with everything. I had always romanticised the idea of meeting my future husband when I was in high school (just like my parents had) and I really thought he was the man I would fall in love with, marry, have kids with and we'd grow old together. He used to see that too, it seemed like the answer, he was wonderful and he thought I was perfect and would tell me every day.

He was my rock through my parents' turmoil, the place I used to run away and hide when life got tough. We spent almost every weekend together and to me, he was my everything, my strength, my protector. There was a time when I dreamed of being a princess and that Ben would whisk me away to his castle where we'd live happily ever after away from drama! And I learned that I got the most attention when I was the damsel in distress and he learned that he got the most praise, love and affection when he was there to save me. What started out as innocent behaviours grew more manipulative after a few years.

His protectiveness became controlling, my desire for his affection became neediness and we started to have this power struggle that turned into regular fights and arguments. But to me that felt normal, we had always fought and it was something I had seen sometimes in my parents' relationship. I thought it was better to communicate and fight while the issue was small rather than letting it build up and not be able to talk, in my mind this was just our way of communicating. What I didn't understand at the time was that it wasn't black and white; that in fact, my parents' marital issues, their fighting and years of tiptoeing around each other was due to not learning to constructively communicate with each other, so then they would implode. To me fighting meant we were communicating but our regular fights became bitter and manipulative, trying to control the other person, which stemmed from our own anxiety around self-worth and the naivety of youth.

In our second year of dating Ben was really struggling with his final year of school, he wasn't getting the marks he hoped for and started skipping classes and smoking weed. That really got to me, Ben had always been against any form of drug and now he was smoking regularly and I thought skipping classes was a ridiculous thing to do.

We spent a lot of our weekends together car shopping because he was about to turn 18 and wanted the perfect first car. One particular weekend we went looking and Ben's dad was with us. We had always had a bit of rough play fighting in our relationship, with a judo background I could hold my own but his parents didn't like it, neither of us knew where the line was that said, 'this is too far'. When we started mucking around that day and he punched me really hard in my arm, corking me. I was in a lot of pain and his dad got really angry with him. I tried to tell him, 'It was fine – it was fine', that it was an 'accident', but his dad told me not to brush it off. Later his parents, who I loved as my own, sat us down and lectured us that it was not OK. It was such an awkward conversation, one I didn't really understand or agree with at the time but I thank them now for doing it.

~ Green and Bitter ~

By the third year of our relationship our lives had changed so much. He had moved out of home so was working to pay rent as well as studying at university. I was in my final year of school then I was planning to take a gap year overseas. I told Ben either he comes with me and we stay together, or don't come and we break up. I was not going overseas for a whole year with a boyfriend back home. He knew I meant it and was afraid to lose me.

We had started to drift apart that year. I was no longer the damsel in distress and had found my voice. Ben was clubbing with the boys and started to question being in a relationship. At one point he asked me if we could be in an open relationship because he wanted to explore what else was out there. I felt so insecure and dug my claws in more. In hindsight we should have gone our separate ways but I think both of us loved the idea of the future we were going to have, the fantasy of it all. And we did have a very strong friendship that served as a good foundation but also made it harder to walk away.

As the year went on it only got worse, we were fighting so much that Ben was banned from seeing me and talking to me during the week so as not distract me from my study and grades. My parents tried telling me that maybe it wasn't the best relationship for me, they saw his controlling side, the side that I thought said, 'I love you'. I didn't listen, scoffing at them, *"What the hell would you two know about a functional relationship?"* Their comments only drove me more into his arms. I felt like they didn't understand me and just cared about me getting good grades. I couldn't wait to run away and have our year together, thinking it would get better.

When school finished, and I was accepted into my first choice for university there was a lot of bitterness and jealousy again. Ben had dropped out of university halfway through the year and didn't really know what he wanted to do, so the fact that I did seemed to really strike a chord. We still went ahead and booked our gap year together, I was excited but terrified. I felt like we were locked into this relationship with matching flights and travel plans for almost an entire year. I did wonder how we would go, but kept assuring everyone that we would be amazing and I still believed we were the perfect match, that we would get married one day and have our family.

I was 18 when we packed our bags and set off for a year, we had to live out of each other's pockets, support each other and face challenges together. We spent our first two weeks in Vietnam, we were in holiday mode and it actually felt like all the stress from home was gone and our relationship had lifted. I looked at my man and for the first time in a long time I felt that deep-seated love.

When we got to England we ended up travelling around for about six weeks to all his family members. While I appreciated their hospitality, I felt alone, this wasn't my family and this wasn't the reason I had come to England. I wanted to work in London, to have fun, not live off Ben's family. I got frustrated with his fear of not finding a job or being able to live in London, he wouldn't even try it. Meanwhile we were spending all of our money on train tickets around England! We started planning ahead and booked to go to Belgium for a family friend's wedding. We would visit my dad in May and we also booked flights to America to meet Ben's biological father in June. While it was exciting it meant we would be living off very little money before we could start work in July.

~ Puppet Strings ~

During a quiet period of our trip, after the wedding in Belgium and a few weeks before we left for America, we were lying in bed when I received a call from home saying my grandpa Eddy was really sick. He had been admitted to the ICU back home and my parents didn't know if he would get through it. I was so torn, part of me wanted to fly back to Australia immediately. I sat up in tears as I tried to talk to Ben, feeling distressed, wondering what I should do.

After a few minutes of my tears he suddenly said, *"I'm so over this."* I sat silently perplexed by what he meant, *"There is always something, your drama never stops. And as soon as it's my turn to get a bit of focus, something else pops up in your life and the attention is back on you."*

I was stunned, *"What on earth do you mean?"*

He glared at me, *"It's just always something Jess, and I need you to be here for me. I am stressed about meeting my dad and this comes up and I feel like I can't talk to you, I can never talk to you!"*

I had tears rushing down my face, instead of love and support I felt like a burden. I couldn't help the timing of this and I didn't know what he wanted me to do. He continued, *"I just don't think I'm in love with you anymore, I don't think I can do this, us anymore."* I felt betrayed and abandoned in one foul swoop, I felt so alone it hurt and my heart ached as I saw the future disappear.

"Please don't say that, don't do this." I begged because I was so afraid to be alone, I didn't understand what was going on and I never thought I would have to do this trip alone.

"Jess I just can't anymore."

I snapped back in anger, *"How can you tell me this, without any warning? I thought we were doing well and this just feels like I'm being backhanded. I am here for you, I've never said you can't talk to me so where the hell is this coming from?"*

He sat there quietly without any answers, eventually he asked, *"Even if we do end this, will you still please come with me to America as a friend?"*

I felt so violated, so hurt, so used, was that the only reason he hadn't said anything before now because he wanted a buddy to lean on in America?

"*No Ben, if we break up then it's over, I will be going to London, I will be doing the things I want to do. I am not coming to America with you, I love you and I will always support you but I can't do that, it will hurt me too much to be with you and not actually be with you.*"

He looked at me like I was betraying him, "*But I need you there.*"

I felt deflated, "*I can't if we aren't together.*"

"*I just don't know what to do, about us, about any of this.*"

I became cold as he tried to hold me, "*Well you have to make up your mind, I am not playing into this.*"

That night he slept on the floor, while I stayed up all night crying and wondering how I had gotten myself into this mess. In the morning Ben decided to leave, he needed some time apart to work it out. He would catch a bus to his aunty's house and wanted me to catch the same bus the next day, once I was there he would tell me his decision. I was lost for words, confused and scared. I didn't want to be alone; to be rejected by the man I thought I loved.

The next day, I dutifully got on a bus for six hours to find out where I stood. To either be told I was loved or that it was over, the ball was totally in his court and I felt sick to my stomach. I got off the bus feeling small and defeated. When Ben met me at the stop he told me he loved me. A smile burst across my face and tears flooded my eyes as I launched my arms around his neck. He apologised and I accepted it.

Letting him back in was another story. I kept him at arm's length, internally questioning him more and unable to really talk to him. Our relationship took a huge step back but at that time, I didn't realise it; I still had him and he loved me and that was all that mattered. I felt myself diminish, I was walking on eggshells, I didn't know who he wanted me to be, or who I should be. Throughout our relationship he had told me I was perfect and now I felt like I wasn't good enough. I didn't understand what had changed, what I had done to change his opinion of me so drastically.

With America coming up we put it behind us somewhat, pretending it never happened. But I felt like I didn't belong, like I should be grateful for him taking me back, that I was lucky he loved me because no one else would. I felt worn down, the spark in my eyes and the spring in my step had gone, I felt self-conscious of who I was, of what I said.

Once in America we seemed to go back into holiday mode, we were exploring a new environment and some of the tension between us eased as we had fun tasting new foods and doing new things. We were having a wonderful trip but ran into an issue when our original plans to go to Florida for a little while at the end fell through and Ben thought it was going to be too difficult and too expensive to go to any of the theme parks. We were flying out of Orlando anyway and I was desperate to go to Harry Potter World, which was nearby. It had been a long-held dream that I had spoken about for so many months and I finally had the chance to go!

When I tried to make plans to make it work Ben threw it in my face that his family had paid for our flights here and that I was being selfish to try and take him away from his family earlier than he wanted. I threw around a few more options suggesting I would still go and he could meet me in Orlando before our flight back to the UK.

"See! You can't stay and support me in what I want, it's always about you, I need you here and I want to stay with my family," he spat back at me.

With tears in my eyes I agreed to put his happiness above mine, to put my dream of Harry Potter World aside because I was scared if I didn't, he would leave. I was losing myself to this relationship, my identity was fading away trying to be who Ben wanted me to be. I was sad about not getting to Harry Potter World but it wasn't about that, it was about how much I had changed. Usually I would have stood my ground, made it work, made a plan. I felt defeated, as though the fight wasn't worth having, I was always going to lose and all it would do was cause a pointless fight and more frustration so what was the point?

The worst part was that I thought it was OK, that it was worth a few sacrifices. What I didn't recognise was that I was being manipulated and controlled. That this relationship had become more and more toxic. To get to Orlando for our flights, it took fifteen hours on overnight buses but I barely spoke to Ben. I felt so empty ... except for the building resentment.

~ Adrift ~

We returned to England about ten days before our birthdays, which were a week apart. For Ben's birthday we planned on visiting his birth town on the coast and exploring around. A few days into our coastal adventure he became quite reserved and angry. We started talking about what's next, I really wanted to go to London and start working there. He was still pushing back against the idea, getting angrier and angrier at me, eventually he turned to me one day and yelled, *"I can't do this, I can't be with you, I just don't think I love you!"*

My jaw hit the ground; he had ripped my heart out again. I was so confused – I had done everything he had asked, I wasn't fighting with him, I didn't even have an opinion anymore because that felt too dangerous. *"So, what was America all about then? Did you just lie to me before we left because you knew I wouldn't go if we weren't together?"*

He looked at me, tears in his eyes, *"I don't know any more Jess, I didn't lie. I just don't think I can do this. I don't want to spend my birthday with you, coming here was a mistake."*

I sat silently, *"Well what do we do from here? Where do we go? I don't want to be here."* I felt lost for words as he got up and started walking towards the door, I panicked, *"Where are you going?"*

He swung the door open and yelled, *"I need time to think!"* slamming the door behind him.

He didn't come back for hours, while I sat in the house angry and unsure of where I stood and not knowing how I wanted to handle it. He came back with his head hung low. He had brought cigarettes and smoked them (not a usual habit), he told me it was my fault, that I caused him so much stress but that he realised he did love me, that he wanted to make it work.

I wasn't taking the blame for his decisions and I told him that. He needed to make up his mind if he was staying or going, I loved him but I couldn't keep this up. I said it was destroying me.

He cried and apologised, he didn't know what was going on but he had decided on his walk that he wanted to be with me still.

I tried to paint a smile on my face at dinner, to maintain conversation but there was an ache in my stomach. Part of me wanted to runaway then, I knew it wasn't going to change but then I thought of the way love and relationships were romanticised in movies. Sometimes people breakup but – not to worry – they'll always their way back together. I remembered the words, 'Love isn't always easy, but good relationships make it through the tough times and get back to solid ground'. That's where we were, wasn't it? Tough times? We were travelling together, living on a tight budget and in stressful circumstances, this was just us toughing it out. If we could get through this, maybe we would be unstoppable. Maybe I just needed to learn to stop being so opinionated, stop pushing his buttons, that's compromise isn't it?

We kept it together, but in the days to follow I became quiet and introverted. I stopped expressing myself and I walked around with the weight of the world on my shoulders. Everything felt like hard work, and even when I tried to be upbeat because Ben was struggling too it didn't last.

Our seaside holiday came to an end a few days before my birthday. I was desperate to get to London, Buckingham Palace was open to visitors and that's how I wanted to spend my day! But when we looked at the train timetable to get there in time for my birthday, we saw it was going to be twice as costly as it would be to go a few days afterwards. So, Ben decided it wasn't worth the expense and promised we would do Buckingham Palace another time. I did agree with him on the finances but it was hard when I felt like I was giving up another day. But Ben promised to make it a special day, knowing his cousin was having a party and we could loop in the celebrations.

My birthday has always been my favourite day... let's be honest 'month' of the year, I have always celebrated in a big way and dragged it out for as long as possible. But this year I felt small, I didn't want to make a big deal of it. We spent the day with Ben's grandparents, who had forgotten it was my birthday. I felt so alone and hurt, like I wasn't important and didn't matter. I was surprised that Ben hadn't reminded them and I spent most of the day crying on the phone to my family, I just wanted to be at home, to walk away. We had been travelling for a little over four months, we had seven more to go and I couldn't see it getting any better. I tried to pull myself together for the party; having fun and pretending nothing was wrong.

A few days later we were on our way to London, to live! I couldn't wait; this is what we had come for! We found a hostel and started living in an 8-bed dorm with other travellers. Within a week we both had jobs and it was all looking up. I didn't feel so trapped, there were people to meet, friends to make, we weren't spending 24/7 together and it was amazing. My spirits lifted as we found our footing and settled in, exploring beautiful London as we went. We weren't spending so much time together and this seemed to help get our relationship back on track, or at least I didn't feel resentment and frustration towards Ben anymore. We were distracting ourselves; back to light-hearted dating.

Ben's job required a lot of long days, he would work 14-hour days and at least five days a week, he was earning great money but it also was taking its toll on him. My job was a lot more fun, the wages were lower but I worked in a bowling alley with the most amazing work mates around. I made strong friendships and I honestly enjoyed my job. Ben on the other hand really wasn't enjoying his work life and felt a little left out. He did become friends with my workmates over time but he started to resent that as well. *"It's not fair, you just make friends so easily and I just feel like everyone only speaks to me because of you!"* He sounded like he was surprised people liked me, and that he felt he was always living in my shadow.

Emotionally I still felt extremely closed off and our relationship was a bit of a rollercoaster. We had massive highs that were exciting, fun and full of adventure. But the lows were getting harder and faster. Whenever we had even the smallest of disagreements, it would end with Ben in my face, grabbing me by the shoulders so I couldn't move and screaming down at me.

The first time it happened I ran away and hid. I was so scared, then he mocked me for crying. His anger seemed to escalate each time it happened, I felt so stupid and worthless but I learned to stand still in front of him because I was terrified of what might happen if I tried to move, talk back or push his buttons further. I would freeze on the spot, trying to stand my ground and not let the horror of the moment overwhelm me.

Each time I would think, 'He's going to take it too far this time, this is when he will just hit me.' I had already visualised putting on the concealer I would need to mask the black eye he was going to give me. I tried everything I could not to push his buttons, keep quiet, be compliant, say nothing, I would try not to speak until spoken to and yet every now and then I couldn't hold my tongue and he would lash out.

One of my new friends told me one day that she admired Ben and I, that we seemed to be really happy. I turned to her and just started crying, *"Yeah sure, in public, but behind closed doors it's a completely different story! I hate him, I hate being around him, he is so angry, he is so grumpy, he screams in my face, he doesn't have anything good to say about me."*

I remember taking a deep breath in realisation, it was the first time I had admitted it or said anything like that out loud. *"Honestly the only reason I am still with him at this point is because we have matching tickets and I am too scared to do this on my own!"*

I still don't understand why I stayed. I think I was so afraid of the unknowns, not just being alone but also what would happen if I did try and leave. His yelling was bad enough if I had opinion that opposed his idea for the day, what would happen if I decided to leave? I let myself be trapped by fear and kept validating the reasons I had for staying. Every time I saw a glimmer of hope, when things were like they used to be I held on to it, thinking that somehow, we could get back to that, even as I lost myself to the relationship more and more.

I still thought I loved him but in hindsight, I loved the idea of him, the idea we had created together. The distance in our relationship was becoming so blatantly obvious there was no romance, no passion, no joy. We still had good times together, but it was more as friends, when we weren't trying to be more, when there weren't expectations. Travelling and distractions kept our minds busy so we didn't have to deal with the emotions of our relationship breaking down.

By the time we reached South Africa in November I was a shell of the old Jess, quiet, spiritless. I had shut myself away trying to be someone I thought Ben could love. I remember my uncle saying to me that my adventurous spirit inspired him. All I could think was, 'How could I inspire anyone, I'm not adventurous, I'm not anything'. I felt so worthless that I believed he was just trying to be nice. My parents were worried about me when they saw us in South Africa, I had gained a lot of weight on our year away but I was also flat and miserable. I had always been stubborn and loud, but by now I believed if Ben didn't like those traits of mine then no one else would either.

I was excited to backpack around South Africa and see the beautiful country I had been born in but I was scared to spend so much time alone with Ben. I had felt safe being surrounded by my family and being on my turf. Thinking of the next seven weeks together made me nervous. Within the first day things had taken a turn after I panicked when a truck was overtaking a car and was driving straight towards me in my lane at about 130km/h! I wanted to pull over and begged Ben to drive, his answer was that I was pathetic. I was so on edge that moments later when I made a small mistake (not big enough to even remember!) he yelled at me to pull over, that I was an idiot who couldn't drive! I hardly drove again for the next seven weeks and when I did I felt timid and useless.

Tensions rose as we travelled. We spent time with my family along the way which was great but there were long days between and so much to see. I remember a few days before Christmas, Ben got really upset with me. I had told him I was excited to give him his Christmas present but this made him angry because he thought we weren't doing presents and he hadn't got me anything. He told me I was selfish and trying to make him look bad, before he stormed out of the hostel. I could do nothing right at this point.

~ Lightness ... Darkness ~

A highlight of our trip was jumping off the world's highest bungee jump; 216m free fall. I grew up horrifically scared of heights; I had a mental breakdown at ten years old when I discovered our hotel room was up on the 34th floor. My family knew about my fear, so months before we left, Dad mentioned the world's highest bungee jump and actually dared me to do it. He even offered to pay if I went through with it, but if I backed out on the platform, I'd have to pay. As soon as it became a dare I had to prove I could do it – I'm only mildly competitive I swear!

I had a few months to talk myself into doing the jump. I told everyone I knew that I was going to do it so the more accountable I would be to go through with it. On the day of the jump, I felt sick, quite prepared to stay on the ground and just watch. Plastered on the walls though were the words, 'Fear is temporary, regret lasts forever', as soon as I read this, it hit home. There was no way I was giving up this once in a lifetime experience just because I'm a little scared, and so I jumped! It was unbelievable, the most exhilarating and strangely serene two minutes of my life!

Ben made the jump too and it was a memorable day for us both. As we kept travelling around and staying with my family in different places, they would often remark what a great couple we made. I always wondered what they were seeing that I wasn't, that perhaps this is what a relationship should look like, maybe I was supposed to be grateful. In all honesty, I know we put on a good front, acting like everything was good while both being torn apart. Our love just seemed to fade and I would have to tell myself, 'I do love him,' in my head.

After about five weeks on the road, Ben told me that he didn't love me — again. I was hurt but even more, I felt defeated. I just couldn't be bothered. I didn't know what to say anymore so I just sat in silence while Ben cried, I was so numb by this point I didn't really know how to respond. I had built my walls so high and I was just waiting for this to happen again. Eventually I said in a broken, hollow voice, *"I guess this means it's over, it's late tonight so let's just sleep on it, you can sleep on the spare bed and we'll make plans as to how we move forward from here in the morning."*

Ben looked distraught, part of me wanted nothing more to do with him, I wanted physical space between us. But seeing him cry, I couldn't just sit and watch him, so eventually I went over and held him. He kept crying but turned to me, *"I'm so sorry, I do love you, I can't do this without you, I don't want to lose you."*

I felt so torn. It was what I wanted to hear but I also felt such relief when I thought about just leaving.

"I don't know Ben, I don't know if I can keep doing this, I do love you, of course I do but I don't know if I can keep being told every three months that you don't love me. Maybe it is best we go our separate ways."

We talked back and forth like that for a while. Eventually we decided to give it one last go, saying that things will get better when we got home.

We reached Sodwana a few days later and went SCUBA diving every day, it was beautiful, blissful and we could see our trip and this rough patch coming to an end. We didn't have the energy to fight and argue and we both loved the diving so it was something to bond over.

The three weeks of diving went far too quickly but goodness me it was beautiful and life changing! In the boat beforehand we would excitedly talk about all the things we wanted to see, about diving, about skills, about decent. But once under water, even though we were all in the same vicinity, you can't communicate, you can only experience the time on your own, see the fish you see, think the thoughts you think. There was occasional pointing by the dive master but at the end of the day the experience you have is up to you, what you are focused on, what you're looking for, your patience.

Back on deck, everyone would talk about their favourite fish or sighting, excited by different things. SCUBA has taught me a very important thing about life, while we were doing the same thing in life at the same time, what we saw and what we experienced was so vastly different, based on our beliefs, on our values and on our focus points.

This period was an amazing interlude from the drama of our relationship. We would be heading home to Melbourne soon; I would start my degree while Ben wasn't sure what he would do. One day back at my aunty and uncle's place in Johannesburg, we were home alone organising and packing to head home. A fight started between us downstairs over something small, I said that I needed some space and huffed back up the stairs. Ben yelled back at me, *"I'm so sick of this drama when it comes to you!"*

I wheeled around, the anger and emotions I had been bottling up for six months ready to burst. I judged there was enough distance (physically and emotionally) that I could say what I liked, so I made a few cutting comments that really got under Ben's skin. Suddenly he stomped towards me in anger, while I was frozen in place. He grabbed me so hard on the arms that I cried out in pain, digging his fingers harder into my skin and he began to scream in my face.

I just managed to wriggle out of his grasp and sprint into one of the rooms. He was right behind me though so I couldn't lock the door. I just pushed it shut and ran and jumped onto the bed screaming, *"Don't touch me! Don't you dare fucking touch me ever again! You're scaring me, you hurt me, don't come near me!"*

He stood at the end of the bed and yelled at me, he was so red in the face. I thought just stay quiet, don't say anything, don't push him further, you don't know how far he will go. I waited it out scrunched in the foetal position on the bed, trying to be small and nonthreatening. Eventually he stormed out of the room; I jumped off the bed and quickly locked the door. I was terrified that he might come back and do something worse. My upper arms were bruised where his thumbs had dug in, they served as a reminder to stay in line, and of the fear that it was only going to get worse.

A while later he knocked on the door to apologise; I told him to leave me alone but he persisted. I could hear him crying and eventually I caved, letting him in but keeping as much distance as I could between us. He apologised over and over again, saying he didn't know what happened, he didn't know why he got so mad, he didn't mean to hurt me. There was always a 'but' though and this time it was, 'If you hadn't poked a sleeping bear and pushed me so far this wouldn't have happened.'

I don't know how or why I forgave him. Possibly it was because I thought he was right. I was worthless and if I was being treated in such a way it was because I deserved it. It probably wasn't really forgiveness as much as giving him his excuses. I gave him every excuse in the book; it's been a stressful year, it will get better when we get home, we will get better when we're home, it won't happen again, he knows it was wrong, I pushed his buttons which I shouldn't have. I took half the blame for his violent outburst; if I weren't such a pain in the ass he wouldn't have lost his temper.

I still felt so trapped. I didn't know who to talk to or what to do, I kept thinking just a few more days and it's all over. I wanted as little do with Ben as humanly possible. I didn't want to sleep in the same room, say the wrong thing, and I also didn't want anyone else to know what was going on because I was scared of their responses. It was hard enough to deal with it the first time it happened, I didn't want to have to talk about it again. I just wanted the last few days with my family to go smoothly and luckily they did.

~ Gone Too Far ~

It was a relief to be home, having my family and friends around me. Ben enjoyed having his mates around too, may of them had become single since we'd left and made comments about him being too young for a relationship. I had so much else going on with starting university and trying to find a job, my relationship took a back seat. We hardly saw each other and when we did we usually fought. It didn't seem to bother me as much because he wasn't the only person in my life anymore. Ben became bitter when I started uni; he hadn't been accepted into the course he wanted while I was starting my dream course studying nutrition and loving it. Ben was biding his time just trying to work as much as possible and I was settling in, making new friends and having a few flirtations with uni boys.

I was becoming independent and finding confidence in myself again. I started journaling again and as a result I wrote a letter to Ben, trying to explain what was going on and what I needed for us to work things out. I held onto that letter, not sure if I should share it with him, would it make things better or worse? One evening as I was heading home from uni, Ben asked to come over. It was last – minute but Mum was great organising us some food. Within five minutes of arriving though, he was angrily storming out. I decided to grab the letter and ran after him, I asked him to read it so we could have everything out on the table. He snatched the letter and stormed away towards his car. I stood behind the open driver's door to try and talk to him. He told me to just fuck off and let him go. When I didn't move he threw his car into reverse anyway and started reversing while I was still standing behind the door. Thankfully I jumped out of the way and slammed the door behind me because I could have been seriously injured if I had moved even a second slower.

After he left, I sat outside filled with fear and confusion as tears poured down my face. An hour later Ben messaged me to say meet him out the front of my house, he wouldn't come inside. I was terrified to know what this conversation would hold. When he arrived I couldn't help but smile when I saw his face, but he couldn't even look up at me, he looked torn apart. When he saw me he burst into tears saying, *"I'm sorry, I'm just so sorry,"* over and over again.

My heart hurt as I saw the internal pain he was battling and my anger and pain fell to the side as I reached out to hold him, *"It's OK."*

He took a step back, *"No it's not OK, I almost hit you with my car Jess! It's not OK!"* I knew he was right, I knew it had gone too far.

"So how do we fix this?" I asked hoping he knew.

"Jess, it's over, I need to walk away, I can't keep doing this to you, I know how much I've hurt you. This isn't me, this isn't healthy."

I was lost for words, I had spent four and a half years with this man, I had travelled the world with him, dreaming of a future, our future and just like that it was over. My reality was shattered, my future felt dark and empty and I scrambled for what I knew, although it wasn't healthy it felt safe, it felt like home.

"It can't be over, it's not over. It's my choice, you can't do this to me, you can't walk away from me!" I cried.

"I can because I know you won't."

His words were like a whip, they stung deep and the consequences of this final decision were overwhelming me.

I was frightened; it was a step in the unknown at the time I never predicted. I thought we were going to be together forever, no matter what. I had never actually thought about a future without Ben, I had spent almost a quarter of my life with him and I didn't remember life without him by my side. I could also hear the pity from people who had been following our trip together on Facebook. So many had said if we could withstand travelling for a year together we could withstand anything. It felt like we had failed.

"I don't want to break up, I don't want everyone on Facebook to know. I don't want all the messages of pity from people I don't care about. Can we just stay in a relationship in Facebook? Can we just work out what this looks like, for us, come to terms with it and then do that?"

When Ben said, *"No Jess, it's really over, we aren't dancing around that fact. Maybe sometime later we will get back together but I think we need some time apart."*

I still asked for one last kiss, but he just turned his back and walked away.

I sat outside, alone in the dark, trying to make sense of this loss, but I was too numb and thought I must have done something to deserve this. Eventually I walked back inside, still sobbing, my eyes red. I didn't know if I wanted to be alone or surrounded with love. I sat up most of the night with Mum, she held me tight and just let me cry.

The next day I couldn't bring myself to eat, everything tasted like cardboard. I still went to uni, trying to keep things moving in a normal fashion, but the whole day I felt like crying, it felt like a piece of me had left. I had tickets for a uni party and Mum told me to go. All I wanted to do was crawl up in a ball but my friends coaxed me into having a few drinks and coming out.

For a moment I did have fun, I felt freedom and a bit of relief as I danced. Later though I was a mess, nothing seemed worth doing if I didn't have Ben, no one else would ever like me; I hadn't even kissed another guy. I sobbed through all of this and one of my guy friends turned to me and kissed me, just to let me know there are other fish in the sea, it comforted me.

I spent that first week in a whirlwind, trying to find myself amongst the mess. I felt more and more like an empty shell. I hardly ate, and hardly slept; I just wandered through life. Ben called me after fours days, to touch base and see how I was going. It was weirdly comforting to hear the voice of the man who had broken my heart. I still felt like there might be a future somewhere on the horizon.

He said he didn't know if we'd get back together, that he didn't promise that, had just said maybe one day. I felt angry and rejected. I was being toyed with again. I found an excuse to hang up the phone and burst into angry tears of confusion. Dad told me I needed to let it go and make him realise that he can't have some of me; it's all or nothing, there is no in-between while he made up his mind. So, when Ben messaged me to organise a convenient time to get his stuff back, I told him to come when I wouldn't be home.

I wrote a letter to him saying thank you for the lessons, the years of love and fun. But also saying that I needed to start putting me first and that in order for me to move on I needed to take a step away from this situation of trying to be friends. I couldn't be in contact so asked him to respect that and not to contact me unless it was actually to give this another go. I closed off and realised that was the only way I could move forward.

After that I reached out to get help from a counsellor, to help me understand what was next. The first thing she did was label me as co-dependent and a perfectionistic, which jarred me at the time. Ouch! If I look back now, I know it was a true reflection of how I was behaving but I just wasn't ready to hear it. In my mind I had come so far, I was independent, I was finding myself again and I felt empowered that I had cut off communication with Ben. Hearing I was co-dependent made me feel pathetic and judged. I didn't trust her, I didn't want her opinions and I decided not to see her again because I didn't feel like she understood me and what I needed. I had spent the last two years feeling small and judged by Ben, so the last thing I needed was to feel that way by the woman that was meant to be helping me move forward. I couldn't see then the difference between identity and behaviour; how our behaviour and mistakes can help us discover who we are and what we stand for, back then I mistook her analysis for judgement.

I started to move forward slowly, working out who I was and what I wanted for the future. As soon as I'd gained momentum and felt some excitement looking forward, I was tripped up when Ben asked if we could talk. I felt awkward and unsure of myself as he came over. I didn't know where I stood, if this was what I wanted. However when we sat down and talked like old friends, the conversation flowed so easily and I remembered why I fell in love in the first place. It was nice and I missed his company.

He made it clear that he wanted to remain friends. Then moments later he kissed me, throwing me completely off track and confusing me more than anything! I didn't know what to make of it and Ben said quite firmly, *"I am not ready to make a decision, I just want to build a friendship."*

I agreed but pointed out, *"You can't kiss me, it sends me mixed signals."*

For the next three months we would bounce around in this friendship zone. Ben would take a step forward saying he wanted more and then he would step back. At his 21st birthday, he told me again that he loved me and wanted to be with me and make it work. Then two days later, he sat me down and said he'd changed his mind! I was firm in my reply, *"That's fine but you cannot keep doing this to me you have to let me go, we can be friends but you can't keep giving and taking your love, it's not OK. This is your final decision."*

I closed off my emotional capacity for him; I was done playing into his games. I stopped making him a priority in my schedule and that really bothered him. I started dating other guys more seriously, looking at them as if they had potential and not just someone to get me through until Ben changed his mind. He started asking me to do more and more things, even just going out for coffee. When I refused he only got more persistent. I felt stronger on my own, I felt like I had mentally and emotionally cut him off.

A few months later I agreed to a relaxed friendly lunch, and it was, until it came time to say goodbye. Suddenly Ben started crying, telling me he'd fucked up and that he missed me. I felt uncomfortable; I didn't know what to do because I didn't see this as an option anymore. I awkwardly said goodbye and left.

I still struggled though, I didn't have a connection with any of the men I dated, the way I connected with Ben. I was also just so terrified of throwing away four and a half years, I assumed at the end of the day all relationships had their challenges and this was ours, this was the challenge we would need to work through. A week later I had a bad bout of tonsillitis and Ben came over to keep me company, buying me soup and looking after me. He told me he really wanted this, wanted 'us' and he begged me to give it a go. I was vulnerable, and so I agreed. But this time it was on my terms, we would date, not commit to the full relationship right away, and then after a few months if things were going well we would reassess.

We started to date and it was great, easy and natural. I thought the time apart had done us the world of good, allowed us to grow up. I felt like a different person, I had found my voice again and I remember saying that to him. He replied, *"I don't think you've changed at all, you still over-exaggerate everything, it's the thing that annoys me the most about you."* It seemed like such a weird, confusing statement that I left it at that.

We never ended up having that chat, to reassess the situation, in my mind it had fluidly settled into place together, we were exclusive and that was it. Then one day just before Christmas 2013, I was sitting next to him and I got a text from Sam from work. I saw Ben's eyes dart towards my screen and I quickly said, *"It's just my friend Samantha from work, don't worry."*

Quite bluntly he responded, *"Even if it was a guy I wouldn't care, we aren't exclusive Jess."*

That was news to me, *"What do you mean by that!"*

"Well I haven't decided if that's what I want."

I looked back at him shocked. Had he been deceptive, or had I been delusional? I didn't really know but I drew the line there and I left. The night after I met a new guy while I was out with my friends, he took a shining to me and Ben's words that we weren't exclusive rang through my head, so I pursued it. I started putting up my walls with Ben again, I decided I was done trying and a few days later while I was on my way to Merimbula on New Year's day, I told Ben I needed space from him, I needed to work out what I wanted.

I had given Ben a shot again because I had invested so much time in him already. Relationships would always be hard work, but this one with Ben just seemed to be pushing me over the edge. I asked myself, why am I giving him so many chances? Why do I keep giving him the benefit of the doubt, when there are so many guys out there who I won't even give the time of day to because I am so fixated on Ben? Maybe it's time to give a new guy a shot, a real shot.

A few days into the holiday I decided to call Ben just to talk but the conversation quickly became heated and I started telling him some home truths. That he had no respect for me or my time, that he was always bringing me down and talking down to me, that he was treating me the way he promised me he never would, he was treating me the way my dad treated my mum!

Then he said it.

"You're the one that lets me walk all over you."

We had reached the final straw, I told him fuck off, never speak to me again or even think about it, it was over! I hung up the phone and deleted his number and his Facebook. This time I knew I was done; there was no going back. I cried but I also felt proud and powerful, like I'd finally stood up for myself and done the right thing by me. He called a week later but I screened it. That was the last I heard from him for a long time.

The next time we spoke, Ben told me he was going through some very hard times. He wanted to mend his past mistakes and so we managed to repair our friendship. I forgave him for all the pain he had caused, I also forgave myself for clinging on to that relationship out of fear. I know the way he treated me was unacceptable and it taught me a lot about relationships and myself. Now with perspective I see that neither of us knew what to do when our relationship started to crumble, we both just kept believing it would get better with time, however when it didn't Ben's reaction was to push away but he wasn't ready to leave and my reaction was to do whatever it took to get Ben to stay.

Our self-worth and futures were so heavily intertwined in our relationship that without it we didn't know who we were or what life was about. At the end of the day we were young, we were good friends and we made poor choices that impacted us both. Though it's hard to look back over this time period I can see how much I've learned and how much I've grown both because of this relationship and since it ended. I will forever hold a space in my heart for him, because he was there for me through some of the hardest times in my life and supported me through it.

This relationship was such a complicated part of my life. Looking back on it using the principles of PATCH has helped me so much to understand how this time became a cornerstone of my strong character today, a strength we have within us all.

Positive: There is a difference between holding onto the past or the future, and a positive mindset. In this part of my life I was creating unrealistic realities and validating behaviours because of them, I was focusing on the small pockets of hope that were becoming few and far between. I have learned to be realistic, looking at right now instead of who we were in the past or who we wanted to be in the future. If I had looked at our relationship without that air of constant hope to get back to where we started I would have walked away sooner.

There are also worse things than being alone, and that's feeling alone in a relationship. It's better to be alone than to settle for a man and a relationship that doesn't build me up, doesn't challenge me and doesn't hold the same values.

Adventure: The adventure was forgiving Ben for all that had happened and forgiving myself for letting this happen to me, for not honouring who I was and valuing myself. Forgiveness is one of the most powerful things I could do, it set me free from the anguish, the pain, and the hurt. It allowed me to accept what has happened in the past and take the lessons to the future. The forgiveness wasn't really for Ben, I know he appreciated it but at the end of the day it was for myself, allowing me to put that time to rest and move on with my life. I think the saying, 'forgive but never forget,' can build resentment. The way I see it is forgive them, forgive yourself and don't forget the lessons you've learned.

Thankful: I am grateful for this relationship, it taught me so much about myself and what I didn't want in a relationship. It allowed me an insight to the red flags and although there was a time where I felt like a shell of a human being it allowed me to build myself back into someone with strong values, beliefs and boundaries, someone I am truly proud of. I know who I am and I will never ever change for another person. I am also grateful that I got to spend some of my life with this man and his beautiful family. Though we had some awful times we shared some great memories and shared some of our most formative years together, we grew up together and I will always love him like a sibling.

Create: I got to create and rebuild myself from the ground up. I assessed my personal values, relationship values, my boundaries and belief systems at such a young age. I realised that by doing that I was setting myself up for a brighter future with stronger relationships both romantically and as friendships. We accept the love we think we deserve. At the start of the relationship I believed I deserved to be loved like a princess, but as time went on and my self-love and self-worth wore down, I would accept and forgive more and more. This was the cycle I was in and it was emotionally abusive.

Honour: To honour myself. It is OK to walk away from a future I thought I had, a future I'd thought I wanted, when I realised that it wasn't realistic. You can have a vision of the future in your mind that is very different to how it actually plays out in real life. It's important to realise that they can be different and not to hold on to what could be but accept what is and decide if that's something you're willing to live with. If it's not love; respect yourself enough to walk away.

If I don't respect myself and set boundaries, no one else will respect me. I can see that I lost myself in this relationship, trying to be someone I'm not to please a man, and that hurt, it's hard work to be someone I'm not, it's uncomfortable and it created so much uncertainty. I will never put my self-worth in someone else's hands again or allow their opinion to change my beliefs and values.

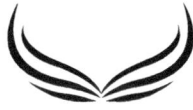

CHAPTER 19

THE PHOENIX RISES....
AND SHE HAS A TEAM MATE

*"Young love is a flame; very pretty, often very hot and fierce,
but still only light and flickering. The love of the older and
disciplined heart is as coals, deep-burning, unquenchable."*
— *Henry Ward Beecher*

One day around May 2017, I realised that my life was back on track, it was amazing in fact. I had overcome most of my challenges and I while I was incredibly happy being single, I felt open to dating and sharing my life with someone. It wasn't the deep-seated need for love and affection I had felt in the past, but more that I had reached a point where I felt whole on my own but ready to explore what else was out there.

I wish I could say from there it was easy. I was terrified; dating had been hard enough without a complex medical background and an eyepatch. While I loved myself I still wondered whether I would find someone who would accept me as I am, who could look past the cancer and see me, rather than a huge red flag. I knew for a lot of people it would be too much to take on. I didn't even know where to begin, I had tried Tinder in the past and I swiped left to that whole experience! I had been out of the dating game for two years and all my friends were in long term relationships so they were very little help in the matter. I had heard a few good things about another app, Bumble, and thought I'd give it a try.

It was hard, with all my photos showing me in an eyepatch there were obviously a few questions, and I wasn't sure how much to disclose. Do I try blunt and upfront revealing that I had cancer or do I play it cool and say it's for medical reasons? I addressed the eyepatch in my bio by saying, 'Pirates wore eyepatches to help them see in the dark, I wear one to get your attention.' While I wasn't embarrassed about my cancer history I didn't want potential suitors to run away before even getting to know me. I had a bit of fun with it, it was nice to be a little flirty and get some attention.

As all online dating goes, most of those conversations went nowhere, until a young soon-to-be-police officer asked to meet-up. Cue panic mode! I was out of my comfort zone just navigating the online world, now I had my first face-to-face date! It was a mild easy date, he was nice enough but our lifestyles were completely different; he was a real boy's boy who loved partying every weekend, I was a relaxed homebody who loved cooking and a glass of wine. I hadn't been clubbing since I'd lost my eye and I didn't plan to get back into it.

While we got along just fine our values weren't in line at all, and when the conversation about the eyepatch came up I was completely honest and told him it had been the cancer, it opened up a whole new can of worms and questions. I felt like I had to share my whole life story with someone I'd known for the space of an hour. I was really uncomfortable; not just revealing my story but I knew he was also judging it to see if there was a future. I decided next time I went on a date I would hold off on opening up about the cancer until I was sure I saw a future dating this man. Although nothing came of that first date, it was a great first step back into the dating scene. There were no expectations for anything to eventuate. It was just a nice one-off date and then we went our separate ways.

A few weeks later, I met up with another guy who I felt a little more connected to at first; he had faced his own physical hardships at a young age and was still thriving in life. I thought he'll understand me a little more, and I didn't feel like I had to hide anything from him being in a similar boat. I picked him up from the train station and chose a restaurant nearby. It was an awkward date right from the get go. As I poured the wine that he'd asked me to bring, he admitted he didn't actually like wine but was drinking it to impress me. To me that meant he wasn't comfortable just being himself but was trying to be someone else in order for me to like him. Our conversation was jagged and filled with awkward pauses. I could see he was a nice, inspiring guy but good golly, there was no chemistry and I felt like I was trying to draw water from a rock, it was hard work.

I had built this guy up in my head thinking we would have so much to talk about and so much in common. I found what we valued and wanted from life was so different. The wine must have given him courage because later on he changed tactics asking to stay over at my house, my family home. I tried to laugh it off but he kept persisting thinking I would change my mind and eventually I had to get quite stern. I felt like he was trying to push me in a direction I was in no way ready for. I drove him back to the station with a thank you and firm goodbye.

When I got home that night, I burst into tears because I was so incredibly conflicted. Although he was great on paper there wasn't any chemistry and I knew I didn't see a future there. But I also felt shallow if I did walk away from him. As I talked it out with Mum, I realised it wasn't about being shallow; my real fear was that maybe that's all I would get. I didn't want to be alone but I also didn't want to settle for just good enough, nice enough. It wasn't about him as a person or his situation; it was the fact that I didn't feel any emotional spark.

~ Matching Maroon Jumpers ~

After that date I felt disheartened, maybe I wasn't ready to date and should just crawl back into the safety of self-love, I was a good enough soul mate. A few days later I swiped right on Bumble to a man who wasn't my normal type, but he had the world's kindest smile and a sassy comment in his profile saying his name is not pronounced 'seen'. He seemed smart, funny and kind so I dove right in replying, 'Surely there's not that many people who don't know how to pronounce Sean, to warrant that comment!' Apparently, you'd be surprised!

After a few weeks of witty banter and busy schedules we tentatively locked in a Sunday date. On the Friday evening I still hadn't heard whether it was on. I didn't realise how hopeful I was until my phone lit up with a message from Sean and I broke into a massive giggly smile. We agreed on a date for Sunday brunch, which is always smart because if the date doesn't go anywhere it'll be over quickly but at least I'll get brunch – the best meal of the day!

On Sunday morning, I was late to wake up and barely had time to shower let alone have a coffee and get all made-up. I remember looking in the mirror and deciding if he couldn't accept me without makeup then he wasn't worth my time, I still can't tell you whether that was pure laziness fuelling that thought or if it were backed by a bit of truth, probably both! I threw on a thick woollen jumper and my jeans and ran out the door not wanting to be late. As I drove past the café I saw Sean making his way inside, just the sight of him set my nerves at ease, he was dressed casually and funnily enough in a jumper the same colour as mine. I didn't know whether that was a little lame but it's still something I look back on and smile.

I strolled into the café a few minutes later and saw Sean was already seated, my tummy flittered with butterflies as I walked over. He saw me and stood up as I walked over, his kind smile lit up the whole room and he gave me a quick hug. I loved how calm and relaxed he was, I was taller than him in my boots and it didn't seem to bother him in the slightest (I had dated a guy previously who used to get upset if I wore shoes that made me taller than him). Sean was comfortable and confident with who he was and I found that incredibly endearing.

We quickly got caught up in conversation and had to ask the waitress to come back several times before we actually looked at the menu. He sat next to me on my blind side, so the entire time I had my head turned at an awkward angle. I didn't want to complain or bring too much attention to the patch or my blind side so I said nothing.

I ordered a double espresso and was incredibly surprised when Sean went for a tea instead, he quickly mentioned he hated coffee and I wondered if we had a future. In the same line of conversation, he mentioned also not liking wine. He had a cheap cask wine experience in uni, I had to hold my tongue so I didn't lecture him about not likening quality wine to cheap goon!

We talked nonstop for two hours, about family, friends, sport, travel, study, work and a million other topics. I really liked the way he spoke so highly of his friends and family, I could see the love and respect he had for them. He also came from a big family; he was the eldest of four kids, like myself and had three younger sisters, the middle of which were twins. We laughed at the fact our family was laid out the same; just the boy in mine was one of the twins! I was excited to have met someone who understood the dynamic of a big family and valued them as much as I valued mine. Eventually Sean had to leave to go to work and neither of us wanted to part ways, I could have spoken to this man for the rest of my day and it felt like someone was prying us apart with a crow bar. He walked me to my car and gave me a hug, I felt so safe and I didn't want him to let me go. He walked away and I wished he had kissed me.

All I could think about was seeing him again! I had never felt such a strong yet easy connection; it excited and scared me at the same time. Later that night I met up with one of my girlfriends. I was still giddy about my date and she teased me lightly. I wanted to deny I was all loved up and even tapped back onto the dating app I had been using to flick through some other profiles.

But all I could think about was Sean. I honestly didn't want to see or talk to anyone else, I really wanted to see where this could go.

On Monday night, I couldn't hold my excitement in, and I asked him out on a second date. It happened again; we sat talking for hours. We had similar values around love, loyalty, honesty, authenticity, family, friends and work which made everything so easy. I also found out he was the world's biggest nerd, he loved his online gaming, regular gaming, board games and reading extreme sci-fi. This time I had to leave for an appointment and Sean walked me to my car and gave me a friendly hug goodbye. The voice of doubt kept into my mind that maybe he wasn't into me, maybe he just thinks of me as a friend? We'd had two amazing dates filled with laugher and conversation and he still hadn't kissed me!

A day later, he asked me out again and we organised a third date for that week! I put together a flawless plan of wearing a rather sexy outfit, a sheer top with a lacey bra that screamed "I'M INTO YOU!" I promised myself that if it didn't land, if he didn't kiss me after this date I was putting him on the back burner. I also vowed to myself that I would open up about the cancer. I knew I wanted this to go further and but I didn't want to blindside him later down the track. I wanted him to come into this with both his eyes open and that terrified me, not just opening up to him but the fact that I was actually scared he would walk away, I really really liked this guy!

That Friday night we sat at dinner for almost four hours, neither of us had other commitments to race off to and it blew my mind that we could talk so freely and easily. He held my hands at the dinner table and even that gave me goosebumps. I wanted to pull my hands away as I started to open up about having cancer, needing to have physical distance there to protect myself. As I told him his face warmed and he listened, he held my hands with such care, letting me open up and not asking me to share more than I was comfortable with.

I told him it had been cancer, that I had lost my eye and that they'd had to close over the eye socket for good. I explained that it had come back but I had been stable for eight months at that point. He stayed calm even though I expected him to run, I even gave him permission, "I understand if this is too much to take on." I struggled to keep eye contact, my focus on the ground.

He gently said "Hey, look at me." I met his eyes and he continued, "Thank you for opening up, I really appreciate it and I am not going anywhere just because of this, it's not going to scare me away."

It was like a weight had been lifted off my shoulders, a huge barrier knocked over. A massive smile gleamed from my face as I felt a new level of trust and respect for this guy. Our conversation continued to flow and eventually after the waitress had come to check on us for the hundredth time we realised we were one of the last tables and they were trying to close.

It was a freezing winter's night outside, amplified by the fact I was barely wearing a shirt! Sean hugged me goodbye and as he started to pull away, I started to think, 'Good golly not even the shirt worked!' He kissed me and it was magical! I couldn't help but smile mid-kiss, I was filled with such joy and hope for us. We spent the next hour kissing and talking in the parking lot of some random Thai restaurant but it was wonderful. I didn't want to leave, neither did he! Eventually after three missed calls from my worried mum, I regretfully parted ways with Sean and headed home, giddy with excitement.

~ More Naked Than Naked ~

I couldn't get him off my mind. I wanted to spend more time in his company, getting to know all there was to know about him, sharing more banter, more laughs and a few more kisses too. Our next date was already locked in for the Tuesday and it was my turn to plan. Knowing he loved beers I decided to take him to lunch at one of the Mornington Peninsula wineries that also brewed their own beers, it was a fantastic way to get to share an experience that neither of us had to compromise on.

After lunch we went back to my place to cuddle up on the couch and watch a movie. I don't recall what it was, I was far more interested in Sean's lips than whatever movie was playing in the background. He was kissing me and gently running his hands through my hair, my eyepatch began to slip out of place. Panic set in, and I pulled away to retie the leather straps. Sean smiled lightly and said, *"You can take it off, I don't mind"* I awkwardly tried to push his comment away and kiss him instead. Not even a minute later though I could feel my eyepatch loosening off again, and I started to feel sick in my stomach.

I hadn't thought about this before, I hadn't really considered what would happen when he saw me with no eyepatch. I had become comfortable in my day to day life without a patch on, and I knew I loved the way I looked but I wondered if he would, I hated that his opinion of me mattered so much to me. Sean wasn't pushy about me taking it off or leaving it on. He just wanted me to be comfortable, so I retied it one more time and hoped that it would stay on ... it didn't. I remember thinking, 'He's going to see you at some point without it on Jess, you may as well get it over and done with. Rip it off like a band-aid and then you'll know, if he can't love you the way you are it's never going to work out.'

My little pep talk gave me the courage to slip it off. I felt so naked, so vulnerable, so scared and so open to judgement. To me this was more intimate than being seen physically naked, and I was ready for him to cringe or stare awkwardly. So when I met his gaze, he had a look of pure adoration that shocked me. He lightly ran his hand over my cheek and without missing a beat said I looked even more beautiful without the patch. My heart melted and tears pooled in my eye. I was overwhelmed by his affection, acceptance and appreciation for who I was and how I looked. I kissed him and said thank you, no other words could form in my mouth and I just felt so much trust, passion and adoration for this gorgeous human being in front of me.

Removing my eyepatch felt like I was throwing away a lot more than just my leather security blanket, it was tearing down the walls and the barriers I had up to protect myself. Sean was breaking them down at a rate of knots and it made me only more intrigued by him. When he left that evening he said, *"Thank you for trusting me, for opening up and letting me see the real you."* My heart skipped a beat as I watched him walk away, I knew he was someone special and that what we had was beautiful.

I couldn't get enough of Sean's company, he made me laugh, he made me smile, and our conversations stretched for hours on end. I spent as much time as I could with him, even inviting him over for my birthday. He arrived with a beautiful bunch of flowers and a cheesy nervous smile. He met the whole family and we played board games together, he fitted in like a dream. But I wasn't surprised; he had a big beautiful family, and three sisters of his own, he understood the dynamic.

That night I decided to bear all, I knew I was falling for him hard and there was still a lot to explain to him. I felt riddled with guilt that I hadn't told him already, it wasn't that I was keeping secrets but I just wasn't ready to be that vulnerable. I told Sean we didn't know if the cancer was gone, I was still being watched very closely and scanned every two months. I also told him that I was potentially infertile because I knew how important having kids was to him. I shared the details of what I had been through, the brain surgery, the relearning to walk, the treatment.

By the end of that night all my cards were on the table and I felt so uncomfortable, so bare, so open. I hated the thought of him leaving but I didn't want him to keep moving forward without telling him every detail. I looked at this man and I knew he deserved the world. When I look back I know I must have loved him even then because I wanted him to be happy whether it was with me or without me. In some way, I was also protecting myself, giving him everything so that if he was going to walk away, if something was too much, he could walk away before I really fell in too deep. As I babbled on Sean just sat there holding the space, allowing me to share everything I had. He held me close and said, *"None of that is going to make me look the other way, I enjoy my time with you, every moment of it and that other stuff, its stuff we can deal with when it comes up."*

My jaw hit the ground, *"You mean none of that is a deal-breaker? None of it?!"*

He laughed at me and simply said, *"No."*

A few days later, I was dozing off to sleep in Sean's arms and he quietly asked, *"Will you be my girlfriend?"* My eyes shot open, I squealed with excitement and kissed him. Honestly with the amount of time we were spending together I thought it was already implied but it was so sweet that he asked. Apparently, my excitement wasn't enough of a response, and Sean awkwardly asked again, *"So will you?"*

I laughed, *"Of course I will you dork!"*

A few weeks later Sean started to tell me that he really, really really, really, really, really liked me. I sat they're patiently waiting for him to tell me he loved me but after a few more dates and still hearing how much he just really really liked me, my patience was maxed out and I turned to him and said, *"I love you."*

He broke out in a massive smile and said, *"I love you too!"*

I just laughed and said, *"I know. You've been telling me for the last week that you really really, really, really, really like me, it was kind of obvious."* He blushed and laughed at the absurdity.

~ A Rate of Knots ~

Our love continued to blossom as we spent more time together integrating our lives more and more. Sean taught me it was safe to be vulnerable. I loved how well he fitted into my life, with my friends and my family; I loved getting to meet his friends and family. Our lives seemed to mesh into each other's quite easily and I could see such a strong and exciting future with this man. Our communication was incredibly open; I know that a lot of that had to do with opening up and being vulnerable about some of the hardest things in my life. Revealing my cancer and potential infertility so early on meant nothing ever felt as big of an issue. I felt I could talk to Sean about anything, ask him anything and I would get an honest answer.

As things got more serious and our future seemed brighter I really struggled between my head and my heart. My heart knew that this was the relationship for me, that Sean was my soul mate and the man I wanted to spend my life with. BUT my head had me running in fear, falling in love opened me up to so much potential pain, so much could go wrong and I was scared. I also wasn't ready to let go of my, 'Miss Independent' identity and as we started to talk about taking the next steps I created these boundaries around me. I cried, I didn't know what to do, this relationship was moving really quickly and I was at times really struggling to keep up with the emotions and the depth of it. I didn't want to lose Sean, I didn't want to take a step back from where we were or the life we were creating together, but I also wasn't ready to let go of my life as I'd known it! I was so conflicted and Sean was so patient and understanding.

There were challenges around my health and the turmoil of emotions rushing through me trying to come to grips with fast-paced love and the changes it meant for my life. Our communication helped us and we were able to go into discussion mode rather than argument mode. We had both been upfront that we wanted a partnership not just another relationship. I don't think either of us truly knew what that meant back then, the extra work, the time, the compromise so we were learning on the job.

Within the first four months we decided to move in together, to take that next big leap once Sean secured a job for the following year. At this point we still lived forty minutes apart and the travel was getting to both of us so it made sense and felt right. I didn't realise how little I knew about compromise until we started living together. Sean first came to live at my family home for three weeks while we were finalising a place to live for January the following year. My brother had to tell me to clear out a drawer for Sean because it wasn't fair that he was living out of his backpack. I reluctantly did so and although Sean would never have asked, his face lit up when he saw what I'd done.

Over the summer we had a trial run of living together while house sitting for a family friend, it went smoothly and we settled in easily together. Our communication improved even more and we grew ever closer. However, as a set of scans came into sight I went on my own emotional hurricane of scanxiety. My life was amazing, I had an incredible partner, my business was taking off as I had just started coaching, we had a lease signed and everything was looking so bright. The scans were like a black storm cloud that had silently floating in to the sky and were threatening to rain on my parade at any second, flushing it all away and making me start from scratch all over again.

I tried to hide this anxiety from Sean, I tried to bottle it up and pretend I was fine but the fear and the anxiety had its grips around me and I was pushing Sean away. He said something about the future, in 30 years or so and I screamed back and said, *"The future is so unlikely – I'll be lucky to hit 30 Sean!"* Tears were tumbling down my face. Anger that was fuelled by the fear of losing everything I had built ran wild through me. I felt helpless and scared. I wanted to cut and run because that was easier, it was easier to make sure I had nothing to lose so if the cancer was back I was already gone.

This was the first time Sean had seen this side of me, this side of being a cancer survivor; the fear, the anxiety, the crippling emotions. *"Don't talk like that Jess, that's not true you've got to hope for the best!"*

"It's the truth Sean!" I snarled back, *"You knew this from the start,*

you knew my future wasn't set in stone!" Sean looked at me defeated, he tried to hold me but I pushed him away. I was scared and insecure, I hated that he was seeing me like this. I wanted to keep my distance as I felt the anxiety pulse through me. Sean's eyes filled with tears, *"Jess, I don't know what to do, I don't know what to say."* Seeing his sadness broke the cycle of anger and I just crawled up in a ball and started sobbing. I felt so vulnerable; up until now I had kept my emotional rollercoaster behind closed doors and now the floodgates opened leaving me exposed.

~ Letting Go and Letting In ~

Setting up our home caused one of the biggest arguments in our relationship. I had all my artwork picked out to decorate our home and I assumed everything would be done my way. I didn't think Sean would be bringing any more than his furniture, his books and his clothing. Boy was I wrong! He had his poster from the footy, a huge signed Ricky Ponting picture frame, a Gandalf artwork thingy to name a few. I told Sean his posters could live in the garage. Up until this point I had never seen Sean mad, but he was fuming, *"Firstly they are not posters!"* he said through his teeth, *"and secondly this is our home, which means my pictures and the things I like, have a right to be up."*

I just looked at him like he was speaking another language, *"But they don't match my colour palette."*

He looked me dead in the eyes and said, *"Too bad."*

I felt overwhelmed with the changes, the move was coming on so quickly and I felt like I was losing 'me' into a 'we'. I felt like it was going to be all downhill from here and soon enough I'd be expected to go to every footy game and know the players in the Western Bulldogs by name! I just burst into tears, it wasn't about the damn posters it was about my fractured identity, I wasn't sure who I was at this point, how I could be both independent Jess and relationship Jess. I didn't think they could coexist in one little body and I didn't want to lose myself to this relationship like I had the in the past.

Moving in together was a whole new ballgame! We argued about a lot more than just the decorating. We were in each other's pockets, arguing multiple times a week. Considering we'd only ever had two full-blown arguments our entire relationship, we were in new and uncertain territory. Trying to learn the ins and outs of living together was a huge adjustment. Sean had lived in a rather messy boy's house and I had lived at home, we were both completely out of our comfort zone and that created a bit of a warzone. We argued over the smallest of things like the chores, the expectations, finances, friends, free time and who knows what else.

The arguments and the yelling scared me; it made me feel so unsafe and took me back to my relationship with Ben. When we fought I needed physical distance between us, I never wanted to be yelled at in my face again but I knew Sean would never do that. Sean wanted to be near me to feel connected. He would try and hold me and I would move away which only upset my darling Sean. It wasn't until one fight when Sean tried to hug me, I told him, *"Don't come near me!"* He didn't listen and without thinking I physically pushed him away, hard. I burst into tears and started shaking. I couldn't believe what I had done, I was so angry with myself and I just couldn't stop saying, 'sorry!'

In that moment, I realised I was bringing issues, fears and beliefs from my past relationship into my relationship with Sean. If I didn't address it I would push Sean and this incredible relationship away for good. From that moment on I have learned that Sean needs closeness when we argue, to remind us that we are on the same team. That our fight is not 'me vs Sean', but rather 'me and Sean vs the problem'.

Sean has been one of the most amazing things that's happened to me, but still it took me a long time to open my heart fully. I was scared of him seeing me, all of me, my fears, my failures, my anger, my breakdowns, anything I had flagged as unlovable and negative I didn't want Sean to see. Those unlovable things were the things I couldn't accept about myself, that I couldn't love about myself, so how could I expect a man, my man to accept me?

Even as we got used to living together, opening up was hard and I was scared about what would happen if I got sick. I didn't want to love him fully because there was a part of me that felt so selfish for taking the most incredible man I knew off the market, and what if I took a turn and he was left with no-one? It wasn't until I attended

Tony Robbins' 'Date With Destiny' and heard a woman tell her story about losing her husband to cancer. She said she wouldn't change their love for the world, but most importantly that she was ready for love again. I needed to hear that to feel comfortable giving that last part of my heart to Sean. To know that even if I wasn't able to be here Sean would find a way back to love, that he could continue to live his life even if I couldn't be by his side.

It was my biggest fear, that cancer would not just rob me of my life but also rob Sean of his — it was a thought I couldn't bear. I have come to terms with my own mortality, but accepting that it wasn't just my life that I was tampering with was hard. I know none of us are ever guaranteed tomorrow but how do you let someone in when you feel like a ticking time bomb? What I had to realise was that I wasn't holding Sean at gunpoint, he had chosen and continues to choose me, to love me despite an unknown future. I had to stop getting in my own way, and in the way of our relationship, I was letting my beliefs hold us back from something magnificent.

I also realised that I wasn't just depriving myself of love and peace and joy, I was depriving Sean of my whole heart and that was more selfish than loving him ever could be. I came home and finally took down those last walls, I let him see all of me, the emotional rollercoaster journey and I let him into every part of my life, every part of me. Since then I have felt more connected to Sean but also freer to be me, I no longer worry that he'll walk away if he doesn't like that part of me because I now know what it's like to be loved unconditionally and love unconditionally.

The other rule we implemented into our house after 'Date With Destiny' was:

"Trade your expectations for appreciations and your whole life will change"
— *Tony Robbins*

We realised the importance of appreciating each other and everything we do. The power of a simple thank you, and the power of allowing each other to feel seen. Thankfully our turbulent time passed by quickly and was fast-tracked with these big personal steps and realisations I had had. With time we learned how to share our space, our chores and communicate and appreciate each other in our new setting. I'd say it takes at least six months to learn how to live with a partner and iron out the creases, but that time in between, those disagreements were worth it. It was Sean and I establishing our new boundaries in a new environment, it was us coming face-to-face with some of our past beliefs that were holding us back. Although it was a challenge we got through it together and it only strengthened our bond.

Sean and I have shared a lot of challenges, they've tested us as individuals and as a team but our love has never been stronger. We are complete opposites; I'm loud, opinionated, emotional, vibrant, leader, spiritual, talkative, passionate and high energy. Sean is calm, grounded, patient, logical, kind, loving, slow-paced, thorough, intelligent. He is everything I'm not and that's where there is such beauty, he evens me out, he calms me down and I motivate him. We bring out the best in each other, we adore each other's differences because they're what make us, us.

I've never felt like I need to change to be loved by Sean, he makes me feel beautiful and feminine, he celebrates me, he also holds me accountable to myself and my values. He doesn't expect me to be anything other than my quirky beautiful self but he knows how important it is to me, to live my life in line with my values. And I do the same for him. We get to be in each other's lives, we get to journey through life together, challenging each other, growing individually and as a team. Sean isn't just my soul mate; he is my teammate, best mate, housemate, playmate, adventure mate.

I am excited every day to wake up next to this incredible man, but I want to acknowledge that I wouldn't have found myself in such a strong beautiful relationship if it weren't for the lessons I'd learned from my past relationships and from my parents' relationship, as well as the time I put into loving myself, discovering who I was, what I wanted from life and from love. I loved myself so much that I was not willing to change who I was at my core, that doesn't mean I didn't need to compromise my behaviours and make space in my life for a glorious man but it meant that I didn't rely on a man's acceptance of me to love myself, my worth is far more than that. Learning to live without letting fear take over has been the most beautiful and empowering experience, I have found the more love I give to Sean, to myself and to the people around me the more love I have to give, I feel so open so generous with my love now. I used to see love as something weak, but now I understand it's the most powerful feeling we can hold, and when we act in love, when we give our love out the whole world around us becomes more beautiful, more abundant.

I know we still have challenges ahead of us, especially around fertility and creating a family. As we explore our options, we will have some incredibly hard decisions to make that will bring up a truckload of emotions. We can only take it step by step but knowing I have my amazing man by my side supporting me through these challenging decisions is amazing. For now, we have so much to look forward to as we work hard on our personal and career goals, and most importantly, our relationship.

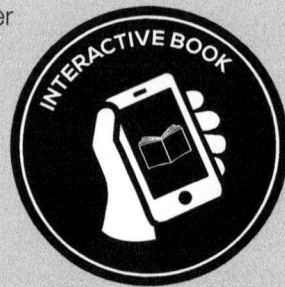

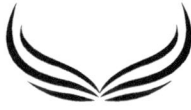

CHAPTER 20

THE UPHILL BATTLE

"Our very survival depends on our ability to stay awake, to adjust to new ideas, to remain vigilant and to face the challenge of change."
— *Martin Luther King Jr.*

My life of adventure, travelling and sport was turned completely on its head throughout those years of diagnosis and rehabilitation, leaving me wrapped in a safety bubble. I wasn't just following the advice from the medical team, this bubble was something I accepted; I was afraid of being alone, being in danger, risking my life in any way after fighting so hard to be here. I was 'strongly advised' to no longer scuba dive or play contact sports like judo.

I was devastated the day I had to cancel my Milford Sound hike, I realised I would be risking my life doing it, that it was beyond my capabilities. It was hard to admit to myself that I couldn't do something, but I found strength in owning it, accepting the hurdle in front of me and promising myself that one day when I was back in full health I would chase this dream.

Gradually as my body got stronger, I started to test my boundaries and wanted the taste for adventure again, not the risky type but anything that wasn't confining me to my own home. One of the first challenges I took on was a high ropes course with my best friend Alanna. It required balance, strength and persistence; it was incredibly fun but also exhausting! I watched as the exhaustion took over my body and my right leg gave way and started to bounce with the familiar spasticity. I learned that day that I could push my body but sometimes it would push back. It was a bit of a game, testing my capabilities, taking precautions and seeing what would happen.

Through the winter of 2017, I flung myself back into skiing, a hobby I had only picked up the year before, it was made even more challenging with a blind side on one side and a weak side on the other. Each turn had its own challenges whether it be the fear of not seeing where I was going down the mountain, or not having the strength and control of my legs and feet. However, my biggest disabler was my very own fear and lack of self-belief.

I had counted myself out of the game, psyched myself out before my skis even hit the snow. I was constantly bracing myself expecting to get hurt, and every fall I had just backed up my belief that because of the situation I was in, skiing wasn't for me. It took a few weekends and persistence and belief from my best friend Alanna to push me out of that mindset and remind me that I can do anything I put my mind to. Yes, I was facing more challenges than your average Joe, but like all things if I held back, if I didn't give it my all, I wouldn't learn, I wouldn't grow! By the end of the winter I felt comfortable to make my turns, hold myself on the runs, get out by myself and enjoy the freedom of skiing. This was the first step in believing that my body was capable of doing things I had loved before!

Over the Christmas period, Sean and I started talking about taking our first overseas trip. I stumbled across a Mount Everest base camp hike and my heart raced. I remembered being inspired at a young age when a classmate's dad had climbed to the top of Mount Everest. I had declared to everyone, *'One day I'll do that too!'* The idea of fulfilling one of little Jess's dreams excited me more than anything. I turned to Sean, *"Would you do it with me? Let's book it now!"* I practically yelled I was so excited jumping around the lounge room.

"Maybe, there's a lot to consider." His calm and logical nature replied. I rolled my eye, getting annoyed that my excitement was met by his nonchalant tone. He knew it was a huge deal and wanted to see the written itinerary. While he went through it with a fine toothcomb (something I mock here but I truly love and appreciate this about Sean) I needed to call Dr Energiser to clear my big idea.

Unfortunately, he ripped the option off the table saying absolutely not! He would not sign-off medically. Not because of the distance but because of the altitude and the risk it would have on my brain, he suggested looking for a hike with lower altitude. After we hung up I was so angry, not at him, but because my dreams were being dangled in front of me but due to my health, they were just far too risky.

For days afterwards, I spiralled downward wanting to throw in the towel. The questions of why me, the despair, the anger, the hurt; I was grieving the loss of not just one bucket list item but half my bucket list. There were at least four other hikes that I had wanted to do that were high altitude like Kilimanjaro and Machu Picchu. There were also all the scuba diving locations I would never see. I had seen a glimmer of my old life but cancer seemed to take charge again. I hadn't really let Sean see me in my lower points but as we'd just started living together it wasn't an emotional rollercoaster I could hide.

I know he felt out of his depths. He suggested that maybe in 10, 20, 30 years I would be OK medically to do Everest, just because it's off the table now doesn't mean it will be forever. I felt so misunderstood, he didn't get what I was going through, maybe he never would. *"Sean, I'll be lucky to be here in five years, at the moment that would be a miracle in itself! Saying that maybe medicine will allow it in 30 years doesn't really help me here buddy! This is something I've wanted for as long as I can remember and now it's not even an option I can consider!"*

I knew that comment hurt Sean; I still hadn't come to terms with my life of constantly being followed by the repercussions of having late stage cancer and what it meant for me both physically and emotionally. I hadn't expressed my fears of not having a future, not being able to see a life beyond the age of 30 because it felt so far-fetched when I was only a little over a year out of my Stage 4 diagnosis. I continued to rant, to weep, to feel sorry for myself for the days to come until on the fourth day it hit me; I had promised myself that cancer would never takeover my life and right now I was letting it take my focus and make me miserable.

~ Not Out ~

With new resolve, I started to search up other hiking options that would be equally as challenging but with less altitude. I changed my focus from what I couldn't do to what I could still do, what life still had to offer. How could I still challenge myself, reach the same level of gratification without hurting myself along the way? I found there were hikes all across the world that piqued my interest and my smile grew. Different reasons prevented many of them simply due to logistics and Sean's work schedule. Then I realised I wanted to find one we could do in the September to mark two years from when I'd taken my first steps learning to walk again. After a few days of looking at all the options, and checking with Dr Energiser we decided we would take on the Kokoda Track. It was listed as one of the most challenging hikes in the world while not having high altitude to contend with. There was also a huge element of Australian history to learn about along the way, which if I'm honest at the time was something that excited Sean a lot more than it did me.

To begin our training, we took on the 1000 steps in the Dandenong Ranges, there were so many people on the track and within a few steps Sean was powering on ahead. By the time we got to the top I wanted to cry, this was such a short hike and even this felt too much for me. I was shaking, exhausted and my leg was bouncing around with spasticity. I wondered if I was biting off more than I could chew, if this was going to push me too hard. I couldn't even hike for an hour without these side effects how was I going to hike for 9 days?!

Sean noticed my attitude change, the contemplation and worry on my face. *"It's OK, we'll get there, we'll train up to it I promise. Remember you did have a serious bout of gastro only 2 days ago!"*

I smirked; I'd been so stuck in my head that I'd forgotten I was still recovering from having my head in the toilet bowel for 12 hours just days before. If I wanted to get through this hike I was going to have to master my mindset, stop the self-doubt, and ask myself how can I do this? What can I do to ensure I am ready in nine months' time?

One of the biggest steps was making the actual commitment; until I had financially locked myself in, it was just a dream. With a bit of research and help from a friend, Sean and I were booked in with Kokoda Spirit. An Australian led tour, which satisfied Sean's want for history and my needs for extra medical support. At this point, all I knew was the hike was about 100km and we would do it over nine days, 12km a day in challenging terrain – that should be fine! Sean had done a much more thorough analysis knowing exactly what we'd be facing and when!

Our serious training started immediately, I wanted to be ahead of the game so we walked or went hiking every weekend and went to the gym during the week preparing ourselves. One of the biggest challenges I faced after overcoming my own mental hurdles, was the doubt thrown in our direction. I had spent a lot of time building up my own self-belief and reminding myself that I was capable of doing it but hearing other people, especially those close to me including my mum, doubting that I could complete the Kokoda track or whether it would be too risky was hard. It caused me to push away from some relationships as a result because their doubt was rubbing off on me. I needed cheerleaders in my life not doubters.

I ended up writing a blog because I was really at my wits' end having to explain to people, both friends and followers why I was doing it and how I knew I was going to do it.

~ Training ~

I was working with an amazing life coach at the time, Gary, who was not only amazing with business coaching but also had a background in trail running and was so insightful. He helped me put a plan together, looking at the event, the Kokoda track date and working backwards looking for milestones and mental ways to prepare. I realised I needed to know I could do a multiday hike at least three months before we left so we booked in dates as well as giving me tips on things like fuelling, training and using hiking poles. Having such a good outline and knowing what I needed to action immediately and what milestones I needed to reach allowed me to focus on moving forward with my goal while building my own confidence along the way.

In the July school holidays, while Sean had some time off, we set off to do a multiday hiking and camping adventure in the beautiful Grampians – this was one of our final milestones. It was just Sean and I in a tiny two-man tent with temperatures dropping below zero every night, the sun setting at 5pm and no running water. Over the three days we hiked about 50km, got lost a few times and learned a lot about how I needed to utilise both my steroids and food. I discovered that my body required regular snacks while I was hiking as well as a decent-sized breakfast beforehand. I needed to increase my regular morning dose of steroids to account for the increased stress on my body and bring forward my evening dose a few hours. I needed steroids to live not to improve my fitness.

I also found out that I couldn't wear sunglasses while I hiked because they impacted my depth perception and ability to navigate steep gradients and rocky ground. We also decided right then, after not showering for four days that there was no way we would be sharing a tent this small in humid Papua New Guinea!

We took on board all that we learned and worked hard the following months as our Kokoda trip crept closer. I struggled a lot with my immune system however, training in winter and having Sean bring home every cold and flu that went through the school he worked at hit me hard, sometimes taking me out of action for two weeks at a time! Although I knew that recovering was important it didn't stop the stress and anxiety building about missing important training days. One of our final hiking weekends was a complete wash-out, there was snow on the roads, lightning and thunder above our heads and sheets of rain coming down. We followed a small circuit that weekend just trying to get the kilometres into our legs without risking being hit by lightning or a falling tree!

My specialists and I had outlined the risks as well as working on back-up plans. I knew I might need to get helicoptered out, or I might need to have a high dose steroid injection. Something as small as gastro could end this whole hike for me. I knew every possible outcome, every possible risk, we had an idea of best-case and worst-case scenario and had to mentally and logistically prepare for every possible outcome!

In the weeks leading up I asked myself what else I would need for the trip. A friend who had completed the track four times had some great advice. He gave me confidence in everything we had packed and organised, he reiterated to take lots of snacks, to go at my own pace, just take it 50 steps at a time. Also, that mindset was everything, something I knew so well but I conceded that in the face of so many new challenges, my ability to maintain my positive mindset may be hindered.

I stepped back and asked myself how I would help my own clients maintain their mindset if they were doing the Kokoda Track. Journaling and practicing gratitude were the first tools that came to mind, but more than that I realised the journaling would need structure, it would ask questions to empower them. The more I dug deep the more I found, and eventually I created my very own mindset journal and hand wrote it for both Sean and I.

The first question was looking for affirmations, 'What do I need to believe about myself in order to keep going?' The answers came from within, 'I am powerfully positive', 'I am ridiculously resilient', 'I am strong', 'I am a thriver', 'I am healthy' and the list went on.

I asked myself for clear answers; why did I decide to hike Kokoda?

1. I want to prove to myself that even after cancer and everything else I have been through, I can do anything I put my mind to and I can still have a full, exciting adventure-filled life.
2. I want my own personal achievements to inspire others to push their limits.
3. I know that doing this with Sean will bring us closer together and show that we can honestly get through anything together as a team.

Next, I asked, 'How do I know I can do this?' The most powerful answer stemmed from my judo training years before when I visualised myself on the podium like I had already won. So my answer here was, 'Because in my mind it is already done! I have watched myself walk the final step; I have celebrated, felt overwhelmed with pride and love'. I know I am completely capable of hiking 93km, it will be tough but I am tougher! I listed off all the amazing things I have achieved like learning to walk again, surviving a disease that should have killed me, that I've learned to love myself through adversity.

The journal also asked morning questions focused around gratitude, love and enjoyment of the day. Followed by the daily rundown, and evening questions focused on lessons, wins and challenges. By acknowledging the emotions of each challenge, this journal would help me maintain my mental strength.

As the weeks became days, we prayed that we had thought of everything, I considered taking spare walking poles but decided against it. On Saturday September 22nd we boarded our flight to Brisbane, massive packs on our back and grins from ear to ear! I barely recognised Sean, his beard and hair were gone, he was clean-shaven and bald. He didn't want to be hot, sweaty and tangled in the jungle. So, me and my bare-faced team mate left.

We would leave for Port Moresby early the next day. In the back of my mind I was worrying about so many things, from my ability to do the hike to what this trip would do to our relationship, would it build us up or tear us down?

I'd seen what an international trip had done to my last relationship, how negative it had turned and while I knew deep down that that wouldn't happen here I did wonder, especially because we would be pushing ourselves mentally and physically! I was open with Sean about my concerns about the fact that I knew he'd need to be watching over himself, building himself up and maybe he'd get frustrated having to wait for me. I was scared I would hold him back. He reassured me, knowing that this trip was just about us as individuals as it was about us as a team.

On our early flight to PNG we met our guide Shane who was travelling with his son. He was a strong ex-army man with a kind heart and I instantly felt at ease knowing he would also be there every step of the way. Slowly over that day we met more and more people that would be joining us on the track, some from other companies, some trekking in the opposite direction to us, and a few people on the return leg of their adventures. Our hotel was an incredible 5-star resort; this would be our last slice of luxury before roughing it on the track for eight nights.

We had a team meeting around the pool to go through everything from what to pack, what we would need and everything we should organise before our departure the next morning. We had a very diverse group; there were nine of us in total ranging in age from 14 to 67, from different states and different walks of life. I was the only female and we were the only couple. We talked about our training and our preparation and by the sounds of it, Sean and I had been training a lot, so we were quietly confident about our ability to get through this challenge.

We sorted through our bags one final time, leaving behind a few things and racing down to the pharmacy to get some extra supplies we'd forgotten or hadn't even thought of! Sean and I enjoyed dinner together and our last dose of romance before we embarked on our journey, surrounded by seven strangers and stress factors that would require us to be best friends and teammates rather than lovers.

~ Step and Slide ~

Monday morning, I was up early to make the most of my final shower, clean water, fresh hair, a toilet that flushes, a real towel! We loaded up our plates from the buffet breakfast, not knowing what the food would be like on the track. We piled into a small bus and departed, leaving for this journey of a lifetime. One of the first stops we made was at Bomana Cemetery located in Port Moresby, which contains 3776 graves — 2346 Australians and 443 Allied soldiers. It was humbling to walk through row after row of headstones knowing that these men had risked their lives for the safety of their country. I paid attention to their ages, most of them younger than me, the youngest I saw was 16! I sat quietly and thanked them for what they had done, while still being a little shocked that war has to happen at all. These men had to overcome many challenges over their time on the track, as would I and thanked them for paving the way.

Our journey would begin at Owers' Corner, the road there was bumpy and gave me bad motion sickness. We met our personal porters, mine was a short man named Stafford, he was quiet with a genuine smile and only wore thongs on his feet! He strapped my bag to his back and soon after taking a few photos under the arches we were lined up to go! *"Ladies first"* they said, and I was right near the front followed by Sean and half our teammates. A few steps in I realised this track was nothing like we'd walked before; it was uncut, unmaintained and there was clay underneath my feet that my boots could not grip onto.

I tried to keep a good pace while battling to keep my footing. I sped up because I could feel people on my tail, I was only 200m in and already holding them up, and I just wanted everyone to go ahead of me. For a moment, I stopped focusing on my footing and the path ahead of me and I felt my feet slide from underneath me high into the air and next thing I knew I was flat on my bum. I felt my face go red and the embarrassment flow through me as I tried to clamber up quickly, the more I struggled the harder it was to get my feet planted and stabilised.

My heart sank when I saw one of my poles had snapped. This hike was going to be a big enough challenge with two poles and it just became ten times harder! Part of me wanted to throw in the towel right then, walk away, I felt defeated just five minutes into the hike. Sean swiftly handed me his second pole and wouldn't listen to my protests. He just smiled and kept walking.

That day only got harder, mostly because I was so down on myself. I fell to the back of the pack pretty quickly after that, I really struggled on the slippery clay and I wondered if I had bitten off too much. My porter caught me at every slip, it was like he knew I would fall before I did! He didn't slip once in his worn-down thongs and yet I was wearing fancy hiking boots and sliding all over the track! The benefits of growing up in the area that's for sure. I got into camp well after everyone else and all I wanted to do was crawl up into a ball and cry. Sean held me, knowing all I needed to hear in that moment was how proud he was of me, that I was doing a great job. Every time I tried to slip into that victim state of woe is me, Sean put his foot down. Not in a mean way, he empowered me and reminded me of my values.

As I sat with my journal, reflecting on the questions I had set, I realised every time I slipped, I apologised, I said sorry. I was letting myself think and believe that I was a burden. If I wanted to stop that I needed to start saying thank you. I needed to live this week in a state of appreciation, find the joy, the good and the beauty in every day, in the challenges I was facing because they were making me a stronger person. This small switch in my mindset would have the biggest impact on my trip!

I wrote my gratitudes for the day in my journal and as was our tradition, Sean and I shared them together before getting into our separate tents. I was grateful for the space because good golly it was humid and my tent was full enough with my hiking pack but the other part missed having him by my side. That night I flipped to the back of my book, a section where I had asked Sean to write me a letter for my tough days.

"Dear Jess, my love, my soulmate,

I love you so much and I am so proud of you for what you have accomplished to get this far. You are the strongest person I know and I am constantly looking to you for the support I know I need. You inspire me every single day and I am so happy to be able to share this amazing opportunity with you. Just as you support me I will always be there to give you all the love and support that you require. We have trained so hard for this and I cannot wait to share that finishing feeling with you. Your strength and drive push me to be the best person I can be for myself and for you.

I love you more than anything else in the whole universe! You make me the happiest man in the world and I know that you will smash this like: YOU ARE THE VOICE, YOU WILL DEFY THE ODDS!

With all my love, your Sean xxxxx"

Reading his words made me smile, made me grateful to be doing this hike with my greatest supporter and reminded me of what I am capable of.

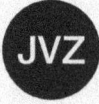

JVZ **Jessica Van Zeil**
5 October 2018
•••

Day 1: Last week Monday on September 24th I started the Kokoda trail with the love of my life and 7 other complete strangers (our guide Shane is missing here).

It's funny to look back at this photo and see the awkward gaps, unsure smiles and very clean clothing.

I remember seeing this group, being surprised that I was the only woman and wondering how we would all mesh! We came from different states, we had completed different levels of training, different reasons for coming to Kokoda, our ages spread from 14 to 67... the only thing we had in common was the goal to finish the track in 8 days' time.

A few minutes after this photo was taken we started heading down the track and within 200m of this starting point I had my first (of many!) slips and one of my walking poles snapped in half. That was the moment I thought "f*ck, what have I signed up for?! Now I have to do this with 1 pole, it was going to be hard enough with 2!" Sean swiftly handed me one of his poles and we continued on our way.

Day 1 was short, we hiked for 3 hours but in that time, I started to realise that this track was tougher, steeper and more slippery than anything we had trained on! I fell to the back of the pack and started to get frustrated with myself, wondering if we'd trained enough, if I was in over my head, if I was going to be holding everyone back.

When I took a step back I realised it would hold everyone up even more if I were to push myself too hard and need to be evacuated out, so stick to my own pace! The other big lesson I learned was to stop apologising for needing help and start saying thank you to the people offering help.

#iamgratefulfor this group of strangers I now call family.

The second morning I bounded out of bed at 5am, after almost 10 hours of sleep! I was ready to tackle a new day with this new mindset, consciously choosing to appreciate every moment, every act, every step of this journey. On the second day, we had two massive climbs and 22 river crossings. I was far more comfortable taking it at my own pace and slowly making my way from spot to spot, taking breaks and eating snacks as I needed.

I could see Sean enjoying being at the front of the groups, bonding with the other men on our trek. While I was glad he was enjoying their company part of me felt a little upset that we weren't really sharing this journey. To my surprise Sean decided to hold back for the last section of the day, walking side by side with me, chatting, laughing and enjoying each other's company. I was so grateful that he took the time to walk with me. I knew I was slow, I was really struggling on the downhills and realised that my depth perception really relied on shadows but under the thick tree coverage it was hard to see. I couldn't judge the distance of a step; I would often over or underestimate my footing. My appreciation for my amazing porter only increased, his patience, his care, his guiding hand down every section, he was incredible and a true lifesaver! I learned to laugh when I slipped and fell instead of beating myself up about it, I found games to keep me mentally stimulated and laughing.

One of my biggest challenges that day was overcoming my preoccupation with, 'The pre-brain surgery Jess would have been at the front of the pack, instead now I'm at the back!' I had to consciously replace those thoughts with how proud the 'Jess in the hospital bed, barely able to take two steps', would be of me now. I reminded myself how far I had come and where I'm going.

I washed in the river that afternoon, taking out my token braids for the first and last time, they were sticky, salty and sweaty, as though I had been swimming in the ocean. That night after our dinner we shared our highs and lows. The men including Sean were very stoic, with a similar response, 'It was a good day, I enjoyed the hike and the views and um ... no lows ... yeah no lows.' Then it got to me and I talked about the incredible highs with a giddy smile on my face and tears in my eyes followed by the lows of learning that the depth perception was such a challenge, I took them on an emotional rollercoaster in my two minute spiel, only to be followed by stoic men again after me.

~ Walk the Walk ~

Within the first few steps out of camp on day three, I managed to slip three times downhill. The path was wet with dew and I was feeling the fatigue all over my body. I wasn't even 100m out of camp when my eyes filled with tears and I just wanted to cry. I was scared I was going to fall and hurt myself, scared that the rest of the day would hold the same for me, slipping, sliding and potential injury at every step. Sean saw me looking defeated and pepped me up telling me to focus on what lay ahead not a few slips I had already had. Sean decided to power ahead on the uphill because otherwise his knees hurt, but promised to stick with me on the way down, no matter how long it took.

Our uphill that morning was three and a half hours of climbing, there were nine false peaks and a lot of laughter as I accurately guessed that our final section was 150 steps and loudly counted as I walked. I found that the excitement and the laughter built up my energy instead of expending it. It kept me excited and my mind busy, not focusing on the strain or the pain of the walk but rather the good things. Once we were at the top I thought the hardest part was over, that it would be a small stroll downhill and we'd be good. Boy I was wrong, the downhill was steep, unstable and I really struggled to step down. I had Sean next to me, but I was so focused on each step, each movement not wanting to plant my foot wrong that I couldn't even speak.

My one eye was constantly having to adjust its focus, and after an hour of this intense movement I started to feel sick to my stomach, like I was going to vomit, it felt like I had motion sickness! So, after a few rest stops to try and gather myself I decided to test out Travelcalm, the same thing I used to combat carsickness. Thank goodness it worked, and although there was still over an hour of downhill scrambling and copious amount of focus, I wasn't feeling like I was going to throw up on top of everything else.

Once we hit the bottom of the valley, the rest of the day involved a flat walk through the marsh and lots of 'bridge' crossings. These bridges were just logs banked up above the water that we had to balance our way over. For one of them I had nine porters helping me get across, ensuring my feet were in the right spot for balance, that I wasn't going to fall or slip. I didn't feel self-conscious about needing help, just grateful that I got it!

We got to see the beautiful sunset from camp that night and I spent some time getting to know the people in my group a little better.

Day 4 was an early start, so early I missed my morning journaling, Shane knew we had a big climb up a mountain face named The Wall! It was straight up, unrelenting and just kept going! I used the mantra I learned at a Tony Robbins event.

"Now I am the voice.
I will lead not follow.
I will believe not doubt.
I will create not destroy.
I am a force for good.
I am a force for God.
I am a leader.
Defy the odds.
Set a new standard.
STEP UP! STEP UP! STEP UP!"

I bellowed at the top of my lungs, it gave me strength and reminded me again that I could do whatever I set my mind to. Apparently, I started quite the stir and everyone in my team wanted to know what on earth I was yelling out! Stafford joined in but Sean was not having a bar of it. He was grumpy and a bit headachy that morning, apparently my yelling did not help that!

We spent most of the day climbing and it was gruelling, by the time we got to lunch it was 3pm. My steroids were low, I had tunnel vision and I couldn't coordinate my steps. I felt so incredibly unwell and stressed. When we reached the lunch stop Sean held me tight and I cried. I couldn't actually speak and that was the first time on our trip I was truly terrified about my health! Sean silently rushed around me bringing me everything I needed. From our many training hikes, he could see my steroid levels and blood sugars were dangerously low. From meds to protein bars to water to food, my plate and my belly was full and all I could do was cry, not because I was sad, or hurt, but because I was scared, and also because that's a side effect of low steroids! My team mates looked on with a bit of worry, this was the first time they'd seen me come into camp unable to bounce around or even smile.

Thankfully after twenty minutes of Sean running around like my personal butler, my medications kicked in and I began to smile again. We prepared for what would be one of the most beautiful experiences of the trip, our memorial service. I'll be the first to admit that up until this point the trip for me was mostly about the personal challenge. I didn't know the history and I had never understood war. I had grown up in South Africa when the apartheid was happening, a hate war that I would never wrap my head around, so to me all war was awful, brutal and unnecessary.

However, to learn that if the battles in PNG hadn't been fought, Australia, as we know it wouldn't be here. Our supplies during WWII would have been cut off and the livelihood of the Australians left behind would be in great danger. The war would have continued down into our beautiful safe country and hundreds of thousands would have been slaughtered or put into war camps. These brave men were fighting to stop that, putting their lives on the line to save their amazing country, the country I am so blessed to call home.

As we stood on Brigade Hill it was hard not to feel the energy of the area, it was one of the most beautiful views and yet in that very space we stood, 87 Australian soldiers had died. We were all asked to read a poem, I cried the whole way through mine. The beautiful men I shared this trip with also cried, it was humbling to see and be a part of. And lastly the porters sang their national anthem, their amazing harmony and love they put into it was breathtaking.

From this point on my trip changed, it wasn't just about me and achieving my goals, but it was about honouring the men who had fought and appreciating all they did for their country. The descent from here was hard and long but I got to spend it with Sean. We spoke about the impact of the memorial service and the poetry that was read. We strolled into camp as the sun was setting; it was beautiful, right on the cliff, it looked like something out of 'Dinotopia'. I took my shoes off as we got to camp, although it was cold I felt the need to ground myself, feel the energy of the track and just get in touch with myself and the nature around me.

That night as we sat around for dinner, our guide Shane told me he had tried hiking with one eye closed. *"The first time I did it, I lasted 10 seconds before I felt off balance and dizzy. I tried it once more and I only lasted 20 seconds."*

He looked at me with pure admiration,

"I knew it was hard for you, but until I tried it I didn't realise how hard. I am so proud of you and your attitude, your ability to keep smiling."

I had tears in my eye, it was humbling to have someone literally take the time to walk in my shoes, to acknowledge my struggles and he then invited everyone else to give it a go. I still have tears in my eye as I write this, because he is one incredible leader!

Day 5 was hump day, the middle day and only involved half a day of hiking! We got to have a bit of a sleep in and saw an amazing sunrise from our little campground. It was weird how cold the nights were getting as we climbed higher and higher. Although this was a short-day hike it was tough, the downhill section we started on had me digging in my bag for travel calm almost as soon as we started. It was steep, and at some sections I felt like I was bouldering rather than hiking! Sean, Stafford and Phil (Sean's porter) patiently helped guide me down this incredibly steep and incredibly slippery section. They were patient and didn't push me to move faster than I could. It was hard and I think it took me twice as long as everyone else but that was OK, today we had time!

When we got to the bottom we had a long walk along the flat, in full sunlight, it was hot and I was lathering myself in sunscreen to protect my skin! Once we got to the bottom of the big climb I felt uneasy, I knew we were going to climb to 2100m above sea level. Shane had warned us of the effects of higher altitude and I started to worry, what if I got dizzy, what if I got altitude sickness even at this height?! Sean could sense my stress and stuck by me.

We took Shane's advice, climbed slowly taking in our surroundings, the views. We sang and laughed and chatted the whole way up. We ran into a few groups moving the other way and I was surprised that the altitude wasn't really affecting me. Three hours later we hit the highest point but then still had to walk along another long flat. At this point it was actually really cold and damp. It was a moss forest, somewhere I could imagine fairies and pixies hiding, it was beautiful, quiet and peaceful. This was a day for reflection and as we walked I realised how surreal it was that such a gruesome war could have happened here. There were lives lost, bombs dropped and yet now as we walked those same trails it was calm and quiet, it was hard to imagine this beautiful place as being a place of fear and terror!

We got into camp at mid-afternoon and it was nice to sit down, relax and just be. I sat next to the running water as I wrote in my journal. I had added extra questions for our reflection day and I felt so at peace, and so proud of myself. I felt like the hardest part was over and the rest was going to be an easier journey to the finish line at Kokoda village.

At the top it was cold, I realised how important those thermals I had been lugging around with me were, the thermals I had laughed at when I saw them on our packing list!

~ Through the Darkness ~

I didn't sleep well that night; I woke up a few times really cold. I felt for our porters who hadn't packed enough warm things! Our adventures started with a detour, out to a spot that barely any hikers got to see, Myola 2. Where the Australians had a supply depot, a hospital and a short runway! The detour was beautiful but meant that we had to hike through overgrown track for the next hour. It was eerie, it felt haunted as the quiet set in and we had to dodge low hanging branches and sometimes lose sight of the people in front as well as the people behind me.

This was a long day and with our detour adding an extra 6 km we were quickly falling behind schedule. Sean stayed by my side again, no questions asked and it was something I really appreciated. It was a day of lots of ups and downs on the track as well as emotionally. I was feeling physically tired but I wanted to keep moving and hitting our targets, but I was falling further and further behind. We got into lunch very late and were told to basically down it and go or we'd be hiking in the dark!

After seeing how much I struggled in the day with my depth perception I didn't want to find out what it was like to hike in the dark. It had become my biggest fear and I was determined to do everything I could to get to camp on time. I picked up my pace and we were walking well, we started playing music on my phone; *The Greatest Showman* of course! We laughed and sang but kept a very determined pace! However, at 4pm, the sun was getting low and the light was making it hard to determine depth, I was really struggling with every step downhill; panic and irritability set in. I had tears filling my eye as I felt like I had done everything I could and it wasn't enough, we hadn't caught up. I felt like a failure as the fear took over my entire body.

Sean grabbed me and with a stern, loving voice told me to not throw in the towel, to keep taking it one step at a time and we'll get there. He told me to keep my chin up, to keep smiling and believe in myself. However, the light was dropping quickly and soon we were reaching for our head torches. I didn't know how far away camp was but night hiking was becoming a reality! We were still about 40 minutes out of camp and my body and my mind went into panic, I was holding back my tears and eventually Stafford took my daypack too. I had three amazing men around me helping with every step. Sean put the music on all over again and it brought a light smile to my face.

We continued moving, about ten minutes away from camp it became pitch black. A few of the porters came up and helped Stafford and Phil with our bags, running them down. Others came up with extra torches and one of the trek leaders, Basil came up and helped me, giving me strong instructions of where to place each foot, every step of the way. That last section that normally would have been ten minutes took us close to thirty minutes. The porters all guided me patiently as I took step by step and held in my tears.

When we got to camp we were greeted with applause and cheers from some of our teammates. Damo was the first one to hug me and I just burst into tears. I was completely overwhelmed with fear and gratitude and pride and exhaustion. Damo just held me in that moment and let me be which is a memory I am forever grateful for.

When Sean got down to the bottom he just held me so tight and told me over and over again how proud he was of me. I looked at my gorgeous man with new sight, he was my absolute rock, my love, my strength when I felt weak, he held me to my values and I realised all over again what an incredible blessing he was to my life.

That special night not only made me feel closer to my gorgeous Sean but the entire team of men around me! I felt protected and loved and I was so incredibly grateful for each and every one of them.

~ Fallen Soldiers ~

The next morning, I woke up feeling surprisingly refreshed. I had faced one of my biggest fears and overcome it. I felt strong, capable and empowered, especially after Shane told us that it was another half-day hike! (let's bear in mind that half day hikes were still from 6.30am-2.30pm). It was a beautiful, slow-paced day filled with laughter, music and an incredible amount of history that I was now lapping up. A lot of our team decided to hang back and see what it was like at the back of the pack, allowing me to lead. They realised at the slower pace we didn't break so much and we got to lap up the beautiful views. Stafford was on my back today, he could see the spring in my step and knew I was clumsy and that could only lead to multiple falls and injury if I got careless! We had a sloped descent, not as steep, nor as slippery as some of the other days which made it enjoyable.

Even after a small hiccup on the road and dealing with a protesting village we got to our campsite in Isarava by no later than 1pm. We had hours of daylight to kill, showers to have (actual running water ... but no heat!). The view from this spot was by far my favourite, we could see all the way out to Kokoda village, it was still 16km away but that was tomorrow's hike. There were mountains, trees, open landscapes. Everyone was feeling bright and chirpy, but also getting hit with nostalgia. I was feeling sad that our amazing hike was nearing the end, it was something I had put on a pedestal and been working to all year and tomorrow it would all be over!

In the later afternoon, we headed down to the memorial site, where four pillars stood that said, 'Courage. Endurance. Mateship.

Sacrifice'. It was the most beautiful spot and the energy was magnetic and calming. We heard the story of the 39th battalion, a group of soldiers who were recruited late into the war and sent over within a day. They had no training, no experience; they were young men most of them in their late teens or early twenties, and most of them died there helping their fellow Australian mates fight. Shane raised the flags and we watched silently, as he stood and started our second memorial service.

Before the readings even got to me I was bawling my eye out. It was incredible to not only have honoured these men with our words, but honoured them by walking the track, by learning about their true Australian spirit and the love they had for the land we will be so blessed to head back to. The poem I read hit me hard and can be viewed in the interactive version of this book. These men, our porters were angels, they were kind and selfless, they helped me every step of the way and they also helped each other, they were incredible and it was amazing to share the track with them.

After the memorial service, we moved to the landing below, we moved silently and sat with our feelings. I moved from the landing to the grass where I took off my shoes and sat with the energy of my surroundings. I looked to the mountaintops we had walked along, to the trees where some of the soldiers hid. It was wonderfully peaceful now but I could almost feel the terror the soldiers fought. I sat in silence and thanked those men, for without what they had done, what they had sacrificed Australia wouldn't be the safe place it now is. Maybe my family wouldn't have moved there, maybe I wouldn't have access to my treatment, to the medical support and the freedom I have back home. I promised that I would never take this privilege of being an Australian for granted, that I would always take every opportunity I was handed and do my work to make Australia even more beautiful.

I thanked them for the legacy they have left. I then asked myself a question that seemed to stem from that, *"If in 12 months I was given just one day to live, what legacy would I want to leave behind me?"* I thought about the main areas of my life. One of the answers was to write this book, I wanted to grow my business so that I could reach and inspire even more people to thrive in their lives. I looked over at my Sean, the man I adored more than anything and realised right then that I wanted to marry him, not just someday down the track but soon!

That was a hard realisation because up until now we had a plan to save for a home, a wedding would come sometime later. This trip and our strength as a couple, as a unit shone through and I realised I didn't want to co-own some house with Sean. I wanted the legacy I left behind in our relationship to be that I was his wife, I wanted to make the commitment and promise to love him forever. I sat in peace with this realisation, knowing it was something I needed to talk to Sean about later.

I struggled to leave my spot on the grass, I felt so connected to this place and I wanted to sit with this beautiful energy all night. Slowly one by one our group headed back up for dinner.

Later that night, we went back down to star gaze on that grass, in that spot. Sean and I sat together just quietly talking and cuddling, connecting on a more romantic note than what we had been all week. I had missed this side of our relationship but the team work and the support we had shared had built up our friendship more than I ever thought possible. Eventually I asked Sean what was most important to him, the house, the marriage or the travelling. He sat silently for a while then said he knew we've always agreed for the house to come first but right then if he could only have one it would be marriage. I sat smiling in his arms and just squeezed him tightly.

JVZ

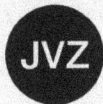

Jessica Van Zeil is feeling **nostalgic** in **Kokoda**   •••
15 October 2018

Day 7 (part 1): Mesmerised

After facing my biggest fear the night before, I was surprised at how easily I got up that day! It might have been the fact we got to sleep in until 5.30am, maybe that it was going to be an early finish.

I was also feeling rather nostalgic, knowing I had just two days left of this beautiful, life changing adventure! Something that we had spent the best part of a year training for and it was coming to an end far faster than I would have liked and I didn't want to waste a minute of it. This was a day filled with lots of war history, beautiful views and fabulous music supplied by one of the porters, Freddy! His favourite song was, 'Keep holding on' by Avril Lavigne and I think we heard it 15 times in the five hours we hiked.

This was one of my favourite days of hiking, it was an easy descent (crazy statement I know!) and a few members of our group hung back and let me lead which was awesome.

We were in camp by 1.30pm which was amazing! It had breathtaking views and a running shower so this was the first time I got to wash my hair all trip.

This photo was taken after our memorial (more about that in part 2). I felt so deeply connected to this place, Isurava. I took my shoes off and sat on the ground allowing myself to get lost in this beautiful place that was once a destination of destruction and fear.

As I sat there I was overwhelmed with gratitude, realising that if this war hadn't been won my family may not have moved to Australia for it's safe and free lifestyle. I may not have received the lifesaving treatment I needed, as Australia is one of the leading countries in melanoma research! I wouldn't have met my amazing Sean and the list went on.

I then asked myself a very important question, 'In 12 months from now, if I was told I had one day left to live, what legacy/memory/ achievements would I want to have accomplished in each area of my life?' I looked at my relationships – with Sean, my family, my friends. My business. My contribution. My health. Adventure ... the list goes on. Some of the answers surprised me and as a result have changed some of my priorities since I've been home.

It's important to remember that NONE of us are guaranteed a long life or even tomorrow but we can have a beautiful life. Stop waiting for next week, next month, next year, next decade to take action towards making your dreams a reality.

#iamgratefulfor this beautiful spot, that reminded me how precious life is and made me re-evaluate what I want out of the next 12 months.

The sun rose between the Kokoda gap, it was one of the most beautiful sunrises I have ever experienced. It would be our last hike, the last day I would have to put my hiking boots on. The last day I would have to worry about my water bladder being full, the last day I would have to ensure I was consuming enough electrolytes, protein, snacks and steroids. I was excited to finally see the Kokoda arches but also on edge, I was loving the disconnection with the online world, just being present and connected to nature and the community around me. I felt sad to leave this beautiful place behind and also a little lost as to what was next when I got home.

I had set my eye, heart and soul on this goal and in a few hours, it would be nothing more than a memory, a past achievement. This goal even eight days ago had felt massive, scary and a little incomprehensible and slowly, step by step, day by day, it had become smaller, closer and more achievable. I could see the finish line and I didn't know if I wanted to get there. The fear of the unknown lay beyond that point.

I slowly packed my bag, and chanted as we went, I got the whole group to do 'Now I am the voice,' chant and it was magical! It was an easy descent, but every hundred metres we dropped the humidity rose and the sun blared down, I watched the most magnificent butterflies fly past, gazed at beautiful views. I wanted to take in every memory, and remember these moments in this place for the rest of my life.

~ Exhale ~

We hit the flat as we came into lunch. I looked back over my shoulder and realised that was it, no more climbing, no more descents, just flat ground from here, it was weird. At lunch, there was a magnificent river, it looked like a pool from a high-end resort ... either that or I was so used to sleeping on floors and swimming in streams that anything nice seemed like a luxury. We sat in the water, talking, laughing and discussing what we would do when we got back to the hotel the next day. The first thing on my list was a shower!

For lunch the porters had made fresh donuts and cut up the most incredible, locally grown pineapples. I can't remember what the actual meal was, obviously the sugar had my attention! For the last section we stuck together, walking as a team, a family. The porters kept darting off into the trees around us and slowly our bags, heads and clothing where covered in flowers and intricately woven crowns. The locals were dressing us up to celebrate and I felt like a queen as I walked with my head held high. I was so proud, excited, overjoyed and overwhelmed. I knew this meant we were almost there.

1 km out Shane stopped us all and unravelled two flags, the first was the Papuan flag. He asked Harold to carry this one across the finish line for his bravery and strength for tackling the track at the age of 67. The second was the Australian flag, Shane turned to me this time. His eyes had a tear as handed it to me, telling me I was brave, that I had displayed the values of a true Australian and of the men who had fought in Kokoda; courage, endurance, mateship and sacrifice. It was an absolute honour to lead our team through the arches holding the Australian flag.

I will never forget crossing that line, the smile that beamed so strongly across my face, the tears welling up and the pride that glowed from the inside out!

The rest of the day was surreal; we relaxed, set up camp, shared a few beers, a few memories and thanked each and every member of our little Kokoda family. We thanked the porters for their hard work and dedication, without them I know I would have struggled to make it to the end injury free! There were tears of joy all around and I cannot thank this magical group of men enough for protecting me, for holding the space, for being there through my laughter and through my tears.

More than anything though I need to thank my Sean, for holding me to my own standards, for being my rock when I needed him, for stepping up and helping me without being asked. For supporting me every step of the way, not just in Kokoda but every single day!

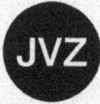

JVZ **Jessica Van Zeil** •••
3 October 2018

On Monday afternoon Sean and I completed our incredible ~96km hike across the Kokoda track.

This experience had been so amazing, it's challenged us both physically and emotionally – I don't know if there was a tear free day but most of those tears were pure gratitude!

It's brought us so much closer as a team and couple because of how often we had to step up to love and support one another through the multitude of challenges we faced every single day!

This trip went far beyond any expectations I had going in and I can't wait to share this adventure with you all in the coming days

#iamgratefulfor every single challenge this trip presented because all challenges lead to growth.

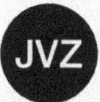

JVZ **Jessica Van Zeil** •••
7 October 2018

Gratitude is the tool that changed my life!

It has been something I make a conscious effort to practice every single day and have for years, yet I'm still astounded at how powerful it is!

On my recent trip to Kokoda I was reminded of this, it was a tough

8-day hike that was both physically and mentally exhausting. The first few days I found myself stressed out, frustrated and full of doubt! I didn't feel like myself. When I took a moment to reflect I realised it was because I wasn't taking the time to appreciate the experience, the challenges, the love, the beauty around me, I was just focused on reacting to the next problem that arose.

It was there and then that I made a conscious decision to be in a state of gratitude for the rest of the trip! It was such a game-changer, I started to consider the challenges as moments of growth, I started to see all the love and kindness around me, I found reasons to smile and laugh. I felt like me again!

#iamgratefulfor this perfectly timed reminder of how powerful gratitude is.

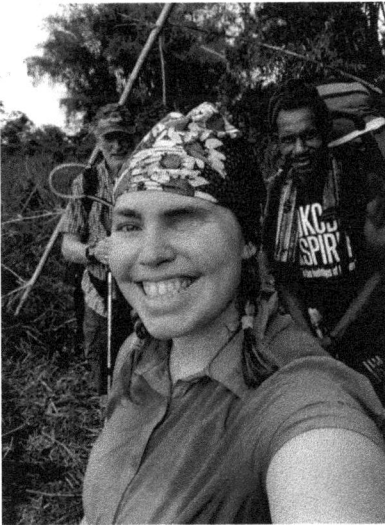

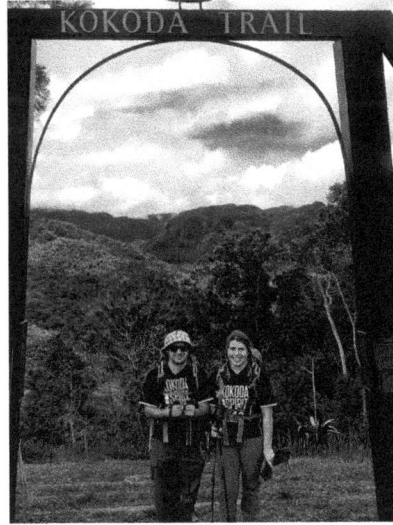

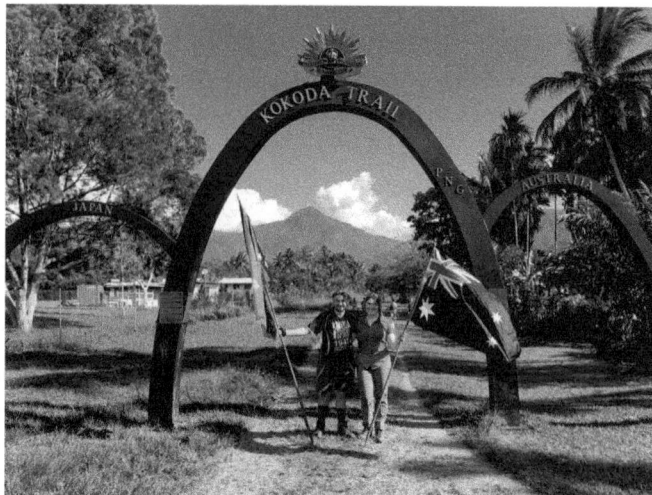

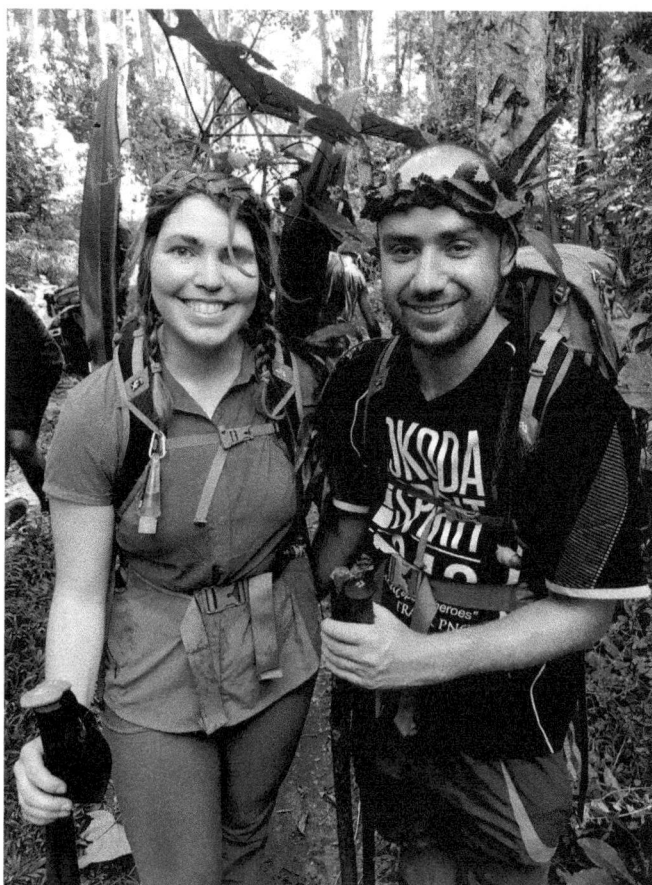

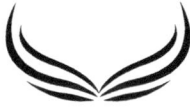

CHAPTER 21

JESS, COACH AND SPEAKER, PLEASE STAND UP

*"I challenge you to make your life a masterpiece.
I challenge you to join the ranks of those people
who live what they teach, who walk their talk."*
— *Tony Robbins*

My first ever speech was at the Melbourne Melanoma March in 2016, I shared my story with 500 people and I shook with nerves as I opened up to them, my vulnerability was obvious. Although I was nervous, I became hooked and continued to find speaking opportunities wherever I could!

Between recovering from the surgery, studying, working and exercising — my neat side-hustle of speaking was taking off and I was one busy girl.

After my interview with 60 minutes, I also spoke at a Victorian Government Youth Summit and other fundraisers, but I was finding myself exhausted and unable to give it my all.

After finishing my degree, I realised that I needed sometime to replenish and just enjoy life. I had spent that vast majority of the last year focusing on my health or my study, so that someday, maybe, I could live the life of my dreams. I realised it was time to focus on me so I could start my speaking career feeling full of life and ready to give my all, not worn down and exhausted.

The next 3 months I spent falling hopelessly in love with Sean, and with life. I put myself first and decided that I was my number one client. By September, I was feeling amazing and felt ready to focus on the future again.

With that decision, I found myself asking "what's next?" — to that, the universe, God or maybe just Facebook algorithms directed me towards Tony Robbins. I had heard his name a few times, I knew Oprah had spoken highly of him and so had my coach, so when the add came up saying he would be in Sydney in a few months, I got excited and clicked on the link. Only to see the price and shut the tab just as fast. Over the next few months I found myself back on the "Unleash the Power Within" website or UPW for short. I was dreaming about going and occasionally wondering over to the website only to talk myself out of it all over again. It wasn't until about 3 weeks before the actual event I found myself back on the site and there was a timer saying ticket prices will go up in 2 hours and I panicked! In that moment I decided, I was going! I booked my ticket, my flights and my accommodation before I had time to reconsider.

A week later, Dad said he would also be joining me because he too had wanted to see Tony Robbins his whole life. Part of me was excited to have someone to go through this crazy event with, the other part was terrified. All I really knew was that I'd be walking on fire and that "life will never be the same AGAIN!"

Yes, at an Anthony Robbins seminar part of the event is firewalking — an ancient ritual practiced through the eras by many different cultures around the world to demonstrate strength, courage and faith. It's a powerful way to overcome fear and take charge of your own mind. As Tony Robbins has said, *"We are trained, almost innately, to be scared of fire and to keep away from it. That is why walking through a pathway of fire is a powerful expression of moving beyond one's fears."*

I got to Sydney feeling a little nervous, was this whole scene really for me? I didn't know anyone besides my dad in a sea of 6000! Within the first few minutes however I had made a whole group of friends, loving every second of it, talking to like-minded people as we danced, laughed and listened. The room had such a high energy to it, filled with music so loud and smiling faces all around me. I felt like I'd found my home, my place, my people! As Tony started to talk about "where your focus goes energy flows goes." I realised I had been using that technique innately when I was training my mind. He spoke about the power of gratitude on mindset, on choosing to be in a powerful state, choosing what will affect you and what won't. I started to realise that the skills and tools I had been using and building — had actual names. And furthermore, I wasn't the only one that believed in them! Happiness *is* a choice.

Getting ready for the firewalk on the first day was powerful. The date of the firewalk landed on was the exact same dates when I had taken my first steps in hospital the year prior. The significance and the reason for doing the firewalk was personal — to prove that anything was possible. That fear would never stop me stepping forward. I walked a full four metres on coals that were a scorching 1600 degrees Celsius and came off with only one tiny blister the size of a pin-head. I felt strong and invincible, high on life!

One of the lessons mentioned at this seminar, was that if I wanted to be the best in the industry, you need to be mentored and coached by the best. My first reaction was "screw you, Tony, it's $2-million to get you for one-on-one mentoring and there is a 2-year waiting list!". He was the best speaker I had ever heard and I wanted to learn from him! But his pricetag was out of reach – for now at least.

I walked away from UPW with a decision to implement 5 changes:
1. Say yes to every opportunity that excites me or scares me.
2. Act on every decision I make.
3. Find a mentor who I trust to help me with the next stage in my life.
4. Perfectionism is a safety-net I hide behind, I will no longer let it hold me back.
5. To believe in myself, in my vision and back myself 100%

Those small shifts changed my life. It altered the decisions I made, the way I felt about myself, the way I spoke to myself and the way I spoke to the people around me. I also reassessed the people I spent time with and if our values were aligned. As a result, I got my website up within a few weeks, started making a business plan, and started taking huge leaps forward in every area of my life.

Within a month I found myself in an audience listening to the amazing speaker, Scott Harris. He was vibrant, authentic, smart, funny, and gave so much value! I listened to him speak and I was on the edge of my seat! When he was done, I went up and introduced myself.

"Hi, I'm Jess Van Zeil and I'm a motivational speaker." I definitely sold myself high, at this point I had spoken at 3 events, but I got his attention. But the truth was I believed that wholeheartedly and so did he, I knew Scott was the man who I wanted to make my mentor and I booked into his 3-day intensive course in late November.

The course rolled around a month later and I sat eagerly in the front row! Deep down I felt a little out of my depth because I was one of the youngest there but I wasn't going to let that stop me. I made a promise to myself that I would put my hand up for every opportunity in the course, to get the absolute most out of it! I got coached by Scott, I spoke on stage, shared my story and had a one-on-one session with him.

I realised that coaching was something I loved, it added a whole new element to my work and allowed me to impact and focus on one person's life. It was something I had always thought of as a career option to add in later down the track, but I quickly realised that those fundamental coaching skills would make me a better speaker too! The only problem was, I had one big hurdle. I had invested all of my savings into self-development already, I was building a business that was hardly off the ground, and my parents and I were recovering from the financial strain of my cancer and my treatment.

When Scott asked me if I was interested in becoming a coach, I burst into tears.

"Why are you crying, Jess?" he asked.

"Because I know this is for me! I have a calling here, but I have explored

every avenue and I can't get a loan as a cancer survivor. My parents and I are still overcoming the financial burden of cancer, I have my HECS debt for my degree, so I am just going to have to put it off for a year, I'm going to have to work really hard, build my speaking business so that this time next year I can say yes."

He held the space with kindness and said, *"OK, I look forward to working with you next year."* I went to lunch and felt a little disheartened that even now, as I tried to make my way in this world, cancer was still finding ways to hold me back.

Our final session for the day was really just a recap of all we had learned, from presenting, to coaching to everything in between and final goodbyes.

As Scott was about to send us off, he made an announcement that he was opening up a scholarship program and they would be taking applications for this program in honour of a young man who had been a part of their coaching program and had passed away from cancer only six-months prior. I felt my heart drop, a deep pang of grief that another young person had faced cancer. But sadly, didn't survive. My heart throbbed thinking of the unbearable grief the family must be going through. But I also felt this moment was a gift and maybe that scholarship was my destiny.

I felt hopeful that maybe I could apply to the scholarship and get in. Then I heard Scott's voice say, *"This year, we have already chosen someone to award this to, and she is sitting in this room."*

My mind was racing, who could it be, maybe it's me, but really could it me, Jess? *"She is a vibrant young woman, a worthy candidate with a bright future, Jess Van Zeil."*

I sat glued to my chair, tears streamed down my face, I was completely overwhelmed by the generosity and the unexpected step forward my life was taking. I gave Scott the biggest hug and thanked him over and over again.

"So, will you be ready to leave in two days?" he asked.

I was lost for words but, *"Yes! I can find my way out of anything I have on!"*

I was drained and super-excited. I had to race home and get my life together to leave, packing for a professional photoshoot and all!

I didn't know what to say when I got home, I was being flown out to the Gold Coast in two days. I didn't have time to get my hair done or anything, I just had to go with the flow, pack my bags and hope for the best! I was a little scared at how fast my life was changing, two months ago I was walking on fire, and since then life had seemed to be full-steam ahead. I was in flow and life was taking me in the direction I wanted to be heading in, all I had to do was make decisions that supported it.

I got to the Gold Coast the morning the course started, I was running late and by the time I walked through the doors everyone seemed to know who I was, Scott had introduced me. I sat in the room eager to learn, but feeling a little out of my depths, everyone seemed so much more experienced than me and I didn't want to disappoint Scott.

Over the next six days, the people in the room became my family, my teachers, and my mentors. We practiced coaching on each other, put our new skills into motion. We had long days, lots to take in, lots to implement, we shared dinners, we shared experiences. Scott took us on his yacht to teach us about dreaming, he set us challenges that pushed us all out of our comfort zone and made us become incredibly resourceful. He prepared us for the next step of our adventure, becoming an actual coach. When we left the Gold Coast it would be our time to shine, to start working with clients and gain experience!

On the last day, Scott asked me what the biggest audience I had spoken to was, I said 500, feeling quite proud.

"How would you feel about speaking to an audience of 2000?"

I looked at him with wide eyes *"it terrifies me a little but I would absolutely love that!"* He smiled and said, *"Good! Because I am working on getting you on a stage!"* I squealed and it was left there.

Later when we got our awards Scott announced to the group I would be speaking on stage in front of 2500 people in May alongside Tony Robbins. *The* Anthony Robbins! My jaw dropped, in less than a year I would go from admiring Tony to sharing a stage with him!

Going home was scary, we had been held closely in the safety of our nest, now it was our turn to jump out and hopefully fly! Within a week however I already had more than enough pro-bono clients lined up and I was ready to commence the next step which was actually coaching. I worked alongside a mentor chosen specifically by Scott to better my skills and become a strong coach who could help make people's dreams a reality. I helped clients build their businesses, their self-confidence, leave their husbands, mend relationships, change careers. Whatever it was they needed to move forward.

Along the way, I continued to engage in personal and professional development, from Date with Destiny, to Scott Demoulin's incredible speakers' program. I've had the opportunity to speak on a wide variety of stages around Australia, finding a love in speaking at schools as well as corporate events.

Sharing a stage with Tony Robbins was an incredible career highlight, I was honoured to share my story with what ended up being almost 6000 people! I was rather scared at first but in the end, I remembered that I was there to help the people in front of me, to inspire and empower them, been scared was only going to hold me back! No way!

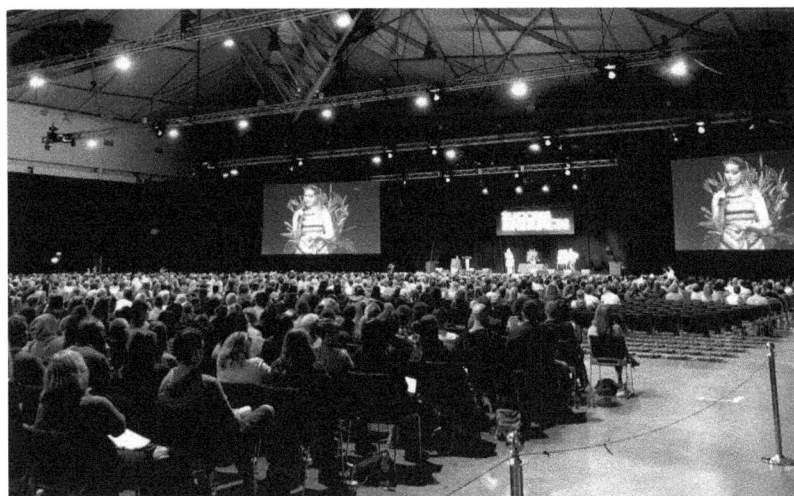

I became a certified coach and I cannot thank Scott Harris enough for believing in me, for taking a chance on me, for making my dreams a reality and investing his time money and energy into me. The lessons I've learned and the people's lives I have been able to change because of him is unfathomable. I thank my lucky stars every day that I invested in myself and believed I was worth it!

I am so blessed to have a career that makes me bound out of bed, one that can touch so many lives and inspire the people to take charge of their lives, believe in themselves and stop surviving and start thriving.

Building resilience is the key to embracing challenges, overcoming adversity and welcoming change. These things are an inevitable part of life and you can either set yourself up to thrive through them, coming out on top even stronger than before, or leave it and scramble to survive.

The course of my life was sailing along a path that I couldn't have imagined, or maybe that's not true! Maybe it's because I did imagine, I did dare to dream, I did dare to stare death in the face and say "No!" that finally my dreams were manifesting before my own eyes.

In a short time, I had found love, became a certified and trusted coach and spoken on some major platforms, even sharing the stage with Anthony Robbins. Surreal.

~ The Word I Never Use Gets the Final Say ~

As I've mentioned, I rarely, if ever, use the word 'perfect' – or I try not to. Perfect is just too...well perfect. It doesn't represent life in all its wild tapestry of highs and lows, peaks and troughs. It's overrated and overused.

But I have decided to make an exception to my 'perfect rule' because something happened one day that was entirely perfect.

Sean and I went to visit his parents in Wodonga. One 'perfect' day we strolled around the Albury Botanical Gardens enjoying the large wise trees, the intimate meandering pathways and the sweet opening of colourful flowers. We took our shoes off and felt the lush grass between our toes. We spent our time relaxing and chatting away. I was telling Sean how much beauty he brings to my life and how grateful I am to share life with him. I was telling him how much his love and support means to me and how I feel we were growing stronger every day.

Sean began to speak, *"I have been trying to plan how I wanted to do this. I got so caught up in all the possibilities, when I realised it didn't matter when or where it was — all that mattered was that I was doing it with you."*

He got down on one knee holding a beautiful elegant ring toward me. I began to cry with surprise and joy when I realised what was just about to happen.

"Jessica Ann Van Zeil, will you marry me?"

I was completely lost for words, tears still racing down my face as I waited for Sean to slide the ring onto my finger as my hands were shaking... it took me a few more seconds to realise the question was not rhetorical and he cannot read my mind.

"Yes!" I threw my arms around the love of my life and kissed him with all the joy and sweetness in the world.

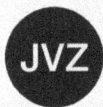

JVZ **Jessica Van Zeil** •••
15 April 2019

#iamgratefulfor the perfect day, in the perfect way with my wonderful fiancé.

The perfect day was the 15th of April 2019. I intend to have many more of them, shared with my soon-to-be husband, Sean.

My post used the word 'perfect' not once but twice.

Though Sean and I have some major obstacles ahead, my fertility issues and wanting a family aren't small topics to conquer together. We want a family, we want to grow old together. So, just as life likes to remind me, it won't all be smooth sailing but the difference is I'm here! I'm happy, I'm alive and I'm in love. I am blessed with the gift of choice. And if I have one message in this book, it's to choose LIFE. To choose your attitude, your mindset and therefore your destiny. You can get through anything with the right tools, you CAN be ridiculously resilient and powerfully positive.

Oh, and don't be afraid of creating your own kind of perfect. It may not be what society deems as perfect or even accepts as 'great'. But you're not here to please society. You're not here to meet crazy standards imposed on you by others. Sean and I aren't perfect but we're perfect for each other. We also work on being the best versions of ourselves for each other.

Perfection is an insane standard if you use it as a comparison. Don't! It's unattainable. You're not here to do that. You're here for a unique reason.

You're here to live fully, unashamedly and boldly as YOU! You're here to shine bright for as long as your life on Earth allows. So, make it count...and most importantly, make it fun. That's what I intend to do. Every—single—day—of—my—beautiful—life. Will you too?

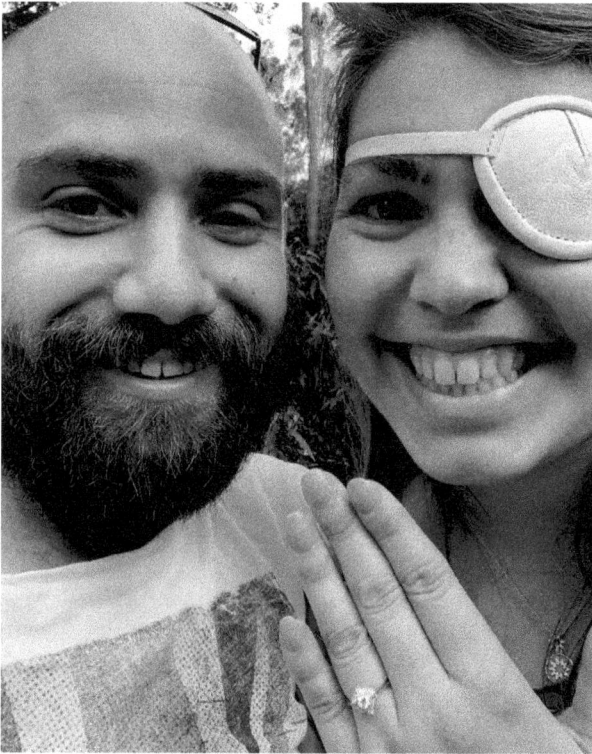

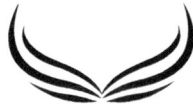

ACKNOWLEDGEMENTS

My big, beautiful family — your support, love and prayers from near and far during some of the hardest moments in my life did not go unnoticed. I appreciate everything you gave up, all the compromises you had to make and that you stood by me even when it was hard.

To my beautiful mum, Heather, you have been by my side every step of the way. I cannot thank you enough for everything you have done, you have been everything I have needed when I need it, my best friend, my carer, my advocate, my protector, my mum. You have picked me up at my absolute lowest points and cheered me on at my highest, I love you to the moon and back Mumma bear.

My incredible dad. I know we have had our rough patches and that I was very much the rebellious daughter who was too stubborn for her own good! But you taught me to use these characteristics as strengths and embrace them fully, without that I wouldn't be the strong woman I am today. Your unwavering support, your persistence and your love is invaluable, and while no one can change the past, I am so grateful for the relationship that we have created, the effort you have put in to get us back to a loving and happy place has not gone unnoticed and I cannot wait for you to walk me down the aisle next year.

Granny Annie, thank you for always believing in us, in what we are capable of and holding us to high standards of love and appreciation. You are such a beautiful, kind and wise role-model and I cannot thank you enough for persisting with your lessons on gratitude, they have changed my life and now will impact so many other lives too!

Grandpa Eddie, I am sorry I never got to say goodbye, but I carry you in my heart always. Whenever things got tough I remembered the strength you showed in hospital and it reminded me that I could get through this too.

My siblings, Britt, Dan and Amy. Wow, what a ride, hey? I am so lucky to be blessed with all of you, you have been patient and understanding, especially when the world seemed to revolve around me, I can't even imagine how hard that was for you. Thank you for visiting me in hospital, for loving on me, for making me laugh and supporting me. I have been blessed with the most amazing siblings that I also get to call my closest friends. I love my tribe.

My friends, good golly, there are too many to name. Thank you for visiting me in hospital, for helping my family, for sharing the load. Thank you for the laughter, the fun, the distractions and the serious conversations. Thank you for being you, my chosen family, the people who didn't have blood ties but showed up anyway, you are all incredible and I am so blessed to have true friends.

To everyone who donated and supported me, your support and love was so incredibly humbling and without you I may not be here. Not only did you help save my beautiful life, but the ripple effect has been massive and the treatment is now on the PBS giving hope to other melanoma patients across Australia. Thank you, thank you, thank you!

To the outstanding doctors, nurses and researchers that impacted my journey, advocated for my case or spent hours upon hours trying to find a cure for melanoma. Thank you doesn't feel like enough, but it's all I have. A massive shout-out to the team at Peter Mac, thank you for treating me like a human being, for bringing outstanding service, facilities and teams to me and so many others. This place was my home away from home, it made me feel safe when everything felt out of place.

And lastly my darling Sean, what more can I say — you got a whole chapter dedicated to you! But in all seriousness, you have been a shining light in my life since the moment I met you. You are my number one supporter, the person who believes in me even when I am filled with doubt, you have held me through the tough times and laughed with me in the joyful ones. Having you here while I wrote this book, my life story, is something I am so grateful for; the amount of tears you wiped away could have filled the bath you ran for me on multiple occasions! I felt so raw and vulnerable through this journey but in your arms I felt safe, like I was at home. I love you unconditionally and I cannot wait to see where life takes us next my gorgeous man.

Lightning Source UK Ltd.
Milton Keynes UK
UKHW041111051219
354823UK00007B/759/P

9 781925 452167